The New Woman's Guide to Health and Medicine

The New Woman's Guide to Health and Medicine

Caroline Derbyshire

*Associate Director
for Consumer Health Education
Women's Care Program
Vincent Memorial Hospital
(The Gynecology Unit of the
Massachusetts General Hospital)
Boston, Massachusetts*

Foreword by
John P. Bunker, M.D.

APPLETON-CENTURY-CROFTS/New York

80 81 82 83 84 / 10 9 8 7 6 5 4 3 2 1

Prentice-Hall International, Inc., London
Prentice-Hall of Australia, Pty. Ltd., Sydney
Prentice-Hall of India Private Limited, New Delhi
Prentice-Hall of Japan, Inc., Tokyo
Prentice-Hall of Southeast Asia (Pte.) Ltd., Singapore
Whitehall Books Ltd., Wellington, New Zealand

Library of Congress Cataloging in Publication Data

Derbyshire, Caroline, 1947–
  The new woman's guide to health and medicine.

  Bibliography: p.
  Includes index.
  1. Gynecology — Popular works. I. Title.
RG121.D44   618.1   79-28121
ISBN 0-8385-6759-2
ISBN 0-8385-6758-4 pbk.

Text design and Production: Judith F. Warm
Cover design: RD Graphics
Illustrations: Sandra T. Sevigny

PRINTED IN THE UNITED STATES OF AMERICA

to my mother,
with love

CONTENTS

FOREWORD

What struck me as I began to read *The New Woman's Guide to Health and Medicine* was that here is a book written by a woman, who is not a physician, telling other women how to take care of themselves. As a physician I was unable to avoid a quiver of concern that important things might be overlooked. I need not have worried. Ms. Derbyshire has invited and received plenty of expert advice. In addition, for almost every situation of any doubt, she tells her readers to "be sure to consult a doctor for advice and treatment."

But could not a physician have written a better guide to health and medicine? I don't think so. A physician could and would have written a different book, certainly, and no doubt a book worth the consumer's attention (there are, of course several such books). The thing about *this* book is that it has something very important to say and it was *not* written by a physician. It was written from the perspective of the prospective patient, and it tells the things a woman should know if she wishes to safeguard her own health and, when she is ill, how to find and use the medical system to maximize her chances of returning to full health.

The message is clear, "Take care of yourself." There are so many reasons to do so! What you, as an individual, do for and to your body has an impact on your health and longevity many times greater than that of the physician. While there is a great deal that you can do, there is relatively little the individual physician can do to keep you healthy; he or she can only try to patch you up once you are sick.

Your role, again as an individual, is equally critical in

determining the success of encounters with physicians and the medical system if and when you need their assistance. It is your decision when to seek help, and whether to accept advice and treatment when they are offered. When the illness or condition is a severe one, and one for which effective medical treatments are available, the decision should be an easy one and can be left with confidence for the physician to make. But much, perhaps most, of the practice of medicine is concerned with less serious conditions, conditions for which alternative treatments may be available, and conditions for which, sometimes, no treatment is preferred by some patients.

When the benefits of treatment consist of the relief of symptoms, and the risks of that treatment include the risk, even the small risk, of death or serious injury, only the patient can make the ultimate decision that the symptoms are sufficiently severe to justify undergoing that risk. We are just beginning to accumulate a systematic body of knowledge on the subject of patients' preferences in such situations, but it is already clear that patients' preferences may be different from those assumed and assigned to the patient by the physician.

In an earlier time the physician usually had an intimate acquaintance with his patients, including a familiarity with their lifestyle and values, and he was probably able to judge with some accuracy what treatment they would prefer, had they the knowledge, in the relatively simple medical decisions faced. Today, the physician–specialist may be encountering the patient for the first time, may therefore have little knowledge of her preferences, and medical decisions are often considerably more complicated and the superiority of benefits to risks less obvious. Under these circumstances, the patient must accept at least a share of the responsibility for her own health. She must be an active and informed participant in the decision process.

But many patients seem to be emotionally and intellectually incapable of accepting such responsibility. One major emotional barrier to the acceptance of responsibility for one's own decisions is regret. If I make a decision that irrevocably alters my future, and if that future turns out poorly, I will always hold myself to blame, I will regret my decision a hundred times a day. If, on the other hand, someone wiser and more knowledgeable than I makes that decision for me; if, in effect, that decision is out of my control, I can perhaps accept the outcome as an act of fate (or, if I believe there may have been negligence, that the physician may have made a bad decision, I may be angry — an easier emotion to live with — and I may even express my anger in a malpractice suit).

That many people cannot, or will not, accept responsibility for their own health is not an insuperable obstacle, however. This is where support groups and social networks can provide essential assistance. Groups of humans, or even pairs of humans, can achieve the knowledge and provide the support for each other that individuals, by themselves, may not be able to. Women, joining forces in a wide variety of health settings have been the leaders in the development of such support services. *The New Woman's Guide to Health and Medicine* is in the best tradition of women's newfound determination to achieve autonomy in health. Its author is to be congratulated for her contribution to the knowledge base available to women engaged in that effort, and for her considerable success in the demystification of the medical care of women.

John P. Bunker, M.D.
Stanford, California
November 1979

PREFACE

"Not another book on women's health care," you may be saying. Yes, but *The New Woman's Guide to Health and Medicine* is different. Times have changed, making this book the outcome of *today's* woman's health care needs. "Very interesting," you may now be saying, "but isn't today's woman capable of dealing with the health care system? Why belabor the point with another book?" If you accept this viewpoint, you will not truly grasp what this book is all about. Although we are over a decade into the women's movement, today's consumer of women's health care services still has to deal with many of the problems that confronted women in the past.

Dr. John H. Knowles, former president of the Rockefeller Foundation, offered a solution to this ongoing dilemma in a bicentennial essay for *Time* magazine on August 9, 1976: "The next major advances in the health of the American people will result from the assumption of individual responsibility for one's own health."

And, that's what *The New Woman's Guide to Health and Medicine* is all about: helping you become your own health advocate. By learning the facts about the sexual and reproductive aspects of women's health care, you — as an individual or through support groups — can take a more active role in the management of your own health.

Organized as a sourcebook, *The New Woman's Guide* provides the most up-to-date information possible on: choosing and using health services, sexuality, sexually-transmitted infections, infertility, and other common health problems. Timely, controversial topics are also covered: birth control, abortion, stilbestrol exposure, surgery, cancer of the reproductive system, breast cancer, and menopause. Most importantly, *The New Woman's Guide* offers specific guidelines on medical problems to help you become an informed consumer of women's health services. By learning the facts, the consequences, and what to do, you can get high quality health/medical care.

But, a book of this nature would not have been possible without the expert advice and support of numerous medical reviewers at the Boston Hospital for Women, Harvard Medical School, The Johns Hopkins Hospital, The Massachusetts General Hospital, New York State Department of Health, Stanford University School of Medicine, University of Chicago School of Medicine, University of North Carolina School of Medicine, University of Washington School of Medicine, and Yale University School of Medicine. To these reviewers, the author is deeply indebted to making *The New Woman's Guide to Health and Medicine* a reality. Responsibility for what is in the book, however, rests with the author.

ACKNOWLEDGMENTS

With many thanks to my reviewers for their invaluable advice and support.

Lloyd Axelrod, M.D., Assistant Professor of Medicine, Harvard Medical School.

John P. Bunker, M.D., Professor of Anesthesia and of Family, Community, and Preventive Medicine, Stanford University School of Medicine.

Thomas H. Green, Jr., M.D., Associate Clinical Professor of Gynecology, Harvard Medical School.

Peter Greenwald, M.D., Dr.P.H., Director of Epidemiology, New York State Department of Health.

David A. Grimes, M.D., Department of Obstetrics and Gynecology, University of North Carolina School of Medicine.

Arthur L. Herbst, M.D., Professor of Obstetrics and Gynecology, University of Chicago School of Medicine.

King K. Holmes, M.D., Ph.D., Professor of Medicine, University of Washington School of Medicine.

Nathan Kase, M.D., Professor of Obstetrics and Gynecology, Yale University School of Medicine.

Rita M. Kelley, M.D., Associate Professor of Medicine, Massachusetts General Hospital.

Ann Kelly, Staff, Boston Hospital for Women.

Richard H. Lampert, Medical Acquisitions Editor, Appleton-Century-Crofts.

Ann Marean, M.S.N., Clinical Specialist in Obstetrics and Gynecology, Boston Hospital for Women.

Jennifer Niebyl, M.D., Assistant Professor of Obstetrics and Gynecology, Johns Hopkins Hospital.

Philip M. Sarrel, M.D., Associate Professor of Obstetrics, Gynecology, and Psychiatry, Yale University School of Medicine.

Robert L. Shirley, M.D., Assistant Clinical Professor of Obstetrics and Gynecology, Harvard Medical School.

Phillip G. Stubblefield, M.D., Assistant Professor of Obstetrics and Gynecology, Boston Hospital for Women.

1

HEALTH CARE:
CHOOSING AND USING IT

Look around, then listen. In conversations, in books and articles, on radio and television, women are saying they want things to be different. This is nothing new. In fact, it has been going on since the late 1960s. Whether active in the women's movement or not, many women have become more aware of their bodies and more interested in the management of their own health. Things were different until the mid-1960s — a time when doctors and their trade organization, the American Medical Association, had almost complete control over the medical profession. Since then, consumer groups have put great pressure on medical organizations and legislators to insure that doctors give their patients more facts about their health plus a bigger say in their treatment.

Out of all this, it has also become much easier to choose and use health services. The media now tell us how to interpret a health provider's credentials to help us make a more informed choice. Indeed, we have come a long way and it all adds up to better health care.

If you know what to look for when seeking health care, it is pretty easy. Here are some basic tips.

But, it is important to know what to expect and what to look for when seeking health care. Here are some basic consumer tips about how to choose doctors, clinics, and hospitals plus what to look for in a good health care checkup.

☐ **DOCTORS, CLINICS, AND HOSPITALS**

Doctors

Choosing a doctor can be confusing. Often, we rely heavily on well-meaning advice from our neighbors, friends, relatives, or even our hairdresser. Sometimes the recommendation works out. Just as frequently, it doesn't. So how can you find a good doctor? Here are some ways:

- Before choosing a doctor, let's get several things straight. Training to be a doctor is a long process. It starts off with earning a Doctor of Medicine or an M.D. degree after completing three or four years of *medical school.* Then comes a year of hospital *internship* under the supervision of licensed doctors in order to become a state licensed M.D. General practitioners, or less than 15 percent of all doctors, generally stop their training here. The remaining doctors go on to complete two or more years of *residency* training in a particular specialty, such as obstetrics and gynecology or internal medicine. A *fellowship* (two or more years) indicates still more training for subspecialties such as gynecologic oncology and endocrinology. All this adds up to nearly ten years beyond college before a doctor is ready to practice medicine. Often, it is longer.
- The most common and easiest way to locate a doctor for your routine gynecologic care, is simply to ask a good doctor you know for a recommendation. Other ways include obtaining a list of "attending physicians" who are on the staff of your nearest accredited hospital; inquiring at a local medical school for the names of faculty members who accept patients; getting a list of doctors from your county or state medical society; or seeking the advice of a well-trusted friend or relative. After you get the names of a few doctors, do some investigation on your own. Use the following checklist as a guide.
- There are essentially four types of doctors who provide routine gynecologic care such as Pap tests, contraception,

and breast exams. Most women use an obstetrician-gynecologist (Ob-Gyn) for their gynecologic checkups. If you want to use another type of doctor for your *routine* care, make sure that doctor can give you the care you need. (For example, not all doctors insert diaphragms and IUDs.) Also — if you develop a problem that your doctor is not experienced in treating — make sure you are referred to a gynecologist for treatment.

Obstetrician-Gynecologist. These are the only doctors who receive long-term specialty training in obstetrics and gynecology. And, in 1976, the Coordinating Council on Medical Education designated obstetrician-gynecologists as "primary care physicians" to women. The primary care physician used to be called the "family doctor." Other types of primary care physicians now include internists, pediatricians, family practitioners, and general practitioners. If you want your Ob-Gyn to attend to your gynecologic care as well as your general medical care, discuss this with your doctor. Make sure your exam includes measurement of your blood pressure, blood and urine tests, plus a general physical exam. (The training program involves one year of internship; three years of residency in obstetrics and gynecology; and two additional years of fellowship training for subspecialties such as gynecologic oncology.)

Internist. Many general internists (specialists in nonsurgical, internal medicine) provide routine gynecologic care in addition to general medical care. (The training program involves one year of internship; at least two years of residency in general internal medicine; and two additional years of fellowship training for subspecialties such as cardiology and endocrinology.)

Family Practitioner. In 1969 the specialty of family practice was created to replace the general practitioner. A family practitioner can meet your routine gynecologic needs as well as your general medical needs and those of your family. (The training program involves one year of internship plus three years of residency in internal medicine, pediatrics, psychiatry, obstetrics and gynecology.)

Moreover, doctors who are Board-certified in family practice only receive certification for a period of six years. For recertification, a family practitioner must pass an exam and submit an audit of their medical activity. Incidentally, the American Board of Family Practice is the only Board which has mandatory recertification, though a few other Boards are nearly there.

General Practitioner. While general practitioners provide general medical and surgical care, these doctors have the *least* amount of training. Generally located in small towns and suburbs, they are rapidly being replaced by specialists. Today, less than 15 percent of all doctors are general practitioners. (The training program involves only one year of internship.)

• Check out a doctor's training. Any licensed doctor can choose to limit their practice to a certain area of medicine without having specialty training in that field. Find out where the doctor went to medical school and did a hospital internship. Also find out where the doctor did a hospital residency and fellowship for further specialty training. A doctor with extensive training at a hospital associated with a medical school is likely to have a solid foundation of knowledge and experience.

Also, check out a doctor's credentials. Find out if the doctor has a license to practice in your state. An M.D. degree alone does not legally qualify a doctor to practice medicine. (In a recent survey, 15 percent of the M.D.s listed in a city telephone directory were not licensed to practice medicine.) You should know the doctor's hospital appointment. If you ever need hospital care, you will be admitted where your doctor has hospital "admitting privileges." Many doctors, especially in larger cities, hold several hospital appointments. The number of appointments is not important but the caliber of hospital is. A doctor who can admit patients to at least one hospital associated with a medical school is most likely to be a good doctor.

• Choose a Board-certified doctor. Though the term "specialist" gets tossed around a lot, only doctors who pass their specialty boards are *real* specialists. Examples of specialties include obstetrics and gynecology, internal medicine, and family practice; examples of subspecialties include gynecologic oncology, cardiology, and endocrinology. Let's say, for instance, a doctor tells you that you have a heart condition. This means you will want a doctor who has at least passed his/her Boards in internal medicine, and preferably, his/her subspecialty Boards in cardiology as well.

Board requirements differ in each specialty. They include a certain number of years of training plus written and oral examinations. This all means that Board-certified doctors must meet established levels of knowledge and standards of practice. For example, one of the things the American Board of Obstetrics and Gynecology tries to do is control unnecessary surgery. Believe it or not, 35 percent to 40 percent of all gynecologists are *not* certified by the American Board of Obstetrics and Gynecology — a statistic comparable with other surgical specialties. Fortunately, noncertified gynecologists tend to do fewer and simpler operations than certified gynecologists.

You can get all this information by calling your county or state medical society. If the doctor is Board-certified, you can also obtain this information from the *Directory of Medical Specialists.* Most public libraries have the *Directory* in their reference section.

• Doctors vary greatly in their opinions, attitudes, integrity, and compassion. Moreover, some are personable and easy to talk to while others are stiff and stuffy. If overall style is important to you, sound out the doctor at your first appointment. Find out the doctor's attitudes toward different methods of contraception, abortion, childbirth, breast-feeding, and so on. Try to see if the doctor is willing to take the time to answer your questions and investigate your problem. Basically, if you don't trust and respect the doctor's attitudes and judgment, find another doctor.

• There are a few things that have little or nothing to do with the quality of a doctor's care. In fact, here are some bad reasons for choosing a doctor:

Social status of the doctor.
Social status of the doctor's patients.
Size of the doctor's practice.
How much the doctor charges. (Some of the best doctors have reasonable fees.)
How long you have to wait for an appointment.
How long you have to wait in the office before your exam.
Membership in social clubs.

Clinics

Whether you know it or not, there are many different types of clinics around. Many are low cost, but some may actually charge you as much as a private doctor. And, according to recent studies, clinics often provide good — if not better than average — health care. Moreover, clinics tend to offer more health counseling and health education than private doctors, and some women use clinics for this reason. But, just as there are advantages to clinics, there are drawbacks. So here are some things you should know:

• There are four types of clinics that provide routine gyne- cologic care as well as general medical care:
Teaching Hospitals. Generally, hospitals associated with a medical school offer high quality care in their outpatient department. Your doctor is likely to be an intern or resident who is supervised by a senior staff doctor. Because these doctors see a lot of patients — many with unusual problems — they are well-prepared to recognize and treat medical problems.
Free standing Clinics. These independent clinics, not associated with a hospital, include neighborhood or com-

munity health centers and family planning clinics. Though originally set up for low-income people, most now accept anyone requesting care. The health care is as good as — if not slightly better than — that in the best hospital clinics. *Public and Community Hospitals.* These hospitals usually offer some outpatient services in their clinic and/or emergency room. (An emergency room is the worst place to go if you don't have a real medical crisis.) Your doctor is likely to be a regular staff physician who also has a private practice. A public hospital cannot refuse to treat anyone because of inability to pay.

Prepaid Group Practice Plans. There are several types of these plans around, though most are often called health maintenance organizations or HMOs for short. A typical HMO offers a range of comprehensive health services from outpatient care to hospitalization. Instead of charging a fee for each service, an HMO collects a monthly or yearly sum in advance from its enrolled members. Right now, HMOs are sprouting up all across the country. The Harvard Community Health Plan, Health Insurance Plan of Greater New York, and the Kaiser Foundation Health Plan are several examples of HMO-like organizations. If you can't locate an HMO in your area, contact the Group Health Association of America or the government's HMO program. (See Readings and Resources.)

- Check out whether the clinic is associated with a hospital, who its doctors are, and their training. Make sure you know the clinic's name and location. For example, is it the general medical or gynecology clinic?
- Ask about the fees in advance and whether you must pay at the visit or can be billed. Most clinics adjust fees according to your ability to pay. Sometimes, fees may be the same as a private doctor.
- Find out if you can see the same doctor each visit. This may be as simple as making your appointment on the same day of the week. Incidentally, unless you have an emergency, make an appointment ahead of time. More and more clinics are trying to discourage "walk-ins" and encourage appointments.
- Find out if the clinic has a transportation service. This

may be important if it is difficult or costly for you to get around. Many of the federally-funded neighborhood health centers and some HMOs have minibuses to pick up and deposit patients.

You can get all this information by calling the clinic secretary or nurse before your appointment.

Hospitals

Every year, one out of ten Americans is admitted to a hospital. Some receive excellent care. Others do not. In fact, about one-third of all hospital patients actually receive substandard care. So, how can you get good hospital care? If you know what to look for, it is pretty easy. Here are some basic tips:

- There are about seven thousand hospitals in the United States that provide medical and surgical care. They can be classified by type of service or ownership. For example, hospitals may specialize in their services, such as obstetrics or pediatrics, or in diseases such as cancer or tuberculosis.

  In broader terms, hospitals can also be classified according to primary source of financial support:

Nonprofit Hospitals. About four thousand hospitals are private, nonprofit institutions, also called charitable or voluntary hospitals. They depend on contributions, endowments, and patients' fees for their support. Within this group, there are teaching hospitals, community hospitals, and religious-affiliated hospitals. Most of the medical profession agree that teaching hospitals have the best services and highest standards. The best teaching hospitals are those that have internship and residency training programs and are associated with a medical school. (Medical students, interns, and residents keep everyone honest and on their toes.) Next best are those with interns and/or residents but without medical school ties. Next in the pecking order of nonprofit institutions come community hospitals and then religious-affiliated hospitals. While some community hospitals are usually good, a sizeable number provide mediocre or substandard care. So, wherever possible, a teaching hospital should be your first choice.

Government-Supported Hospitals. About two thousand hospitals are public hospitals. These include military, Veterans Administration, Public Health Service, state, county, and city hospitals. They are tax-supported and medical care is free of charge to qualified patients. Many government-supported hospitals are affiliated with medical schools and provide high quality medical care.

Profit Hospitals. Of the remaining institutions, about one thousand are profit, private hospitals, also called proprietary. They are owned and operated for profit by individuals or stockholders. In fact, many of the owners are doctors who admit their own private patients to the hospital. Studies show that these hospitals deliver the worst caliber of care. Most are small, having fewer than one hundred beds. With one or two exceptions, they are not affiliated with a medical school. Often these hospitals specialize in a profitable service, such as psychiatric care or simple surgical procedures. While many are poorly equipped, there are a few good ones around.

- Make sure your doctor or clinic can admit you to at least one good hospital. No matter how many good hospitals there may be in your area, unless the doctor has "admitting privileges" to one of them, they are of no benefit to you.
- Find out what kinds of doctors are on the hospital staff. If most of the doctors are Board-certified, you can be assured that high quality medicine is being practiced in the hospital. Also, if there are a wide variety of medical and surgical specialists on the staff, the hospital can provide more comprehensive services. (Just about all doctors on the staff of a teaching hospital are Board-certified.)
- No matter what type of hospital you enter, make sure it is accredited by the Joint Commission on Accreditation of

Hospitals. The Commission is composed of representatives of the American College of Surgeons, the American College of Physicians, the American Hospital Association, and the American Medical Association. Only accredited hospitals are eligible to participate in the Medicare program and receive funds for internship, residency, and nurses' training programs. Since hospital standards do not have to be especially high to receive accreditation, you should avoid nonaccredited hospitals. By the way, about one out of four hospitals is *not* accredited.

• If possible, choose a larger hospital and avoid those with less than one hundred beds. Larger hospitals usually have a wider array of services and can do these well. While there are a few good small hospitals around, most cannot compete with the larger ones when it comes to providing services.

• A good hospital should also have a patient advocate program. Patient advocates — independent of hospital administration, doctors, and other hospital staff — deal with patient complaints and also solicit criticisms.

You can get this information by calling the hospital's administrative office. Or, you can get just about all this information from the *American Hospital Association's Guide to the Health Care Field.* Most public libraries have the *Guide* in their reference section.

☐ **HEALTH CARE CHECKUPS**

What happened during your last checkup? Did your doctor ask about your overall health, check your blood pressure, examine your breasts, and take a Pap test? In other words, do you have a doctor who can meet both your general health needs as well as your gynecologic needs? Or, do you have to make two appointments, one with an internist or family practitioner and another with a gynecologist? Whatever your situation may be, get regular checkups for your overall health care. How often you need to have checkups varies from woman to woman. Usually all women over eighteen should have a checkup exam with a Pap test once a year. But, ask your doctor how often you should schedule these exams.

Good health care checkups include:

Medical History

Your first visit to a new doctor or clinic should include questions about you and your family's past and present health. (See Table 1, pages 18-19) Called the "medical history," it is the single most important part of any exam. This is because it gives your doctor a complete picture of your general health, possible hereditary tendencies (many health problems tend to run in families), and diagnosis of a problem if you have one. It also gives you a chance to speak up about any problems that may be bothering you. (Make it a point to be specific when you describe your symptoms.) There are several ways your doctor can gather this information. Usually the doctor takes your history before your exam. But some doctors and clinics have you fill out a form before you talk to the doctor. Or your medical history and exam may be done by the doctor's assistant. In fact, more and more doctors now use specially-trained assistants, such as a nurse practitioner, for routine histories and exams.

A good medical history takes time. Surprisingly, a number of doctors spend only a few minutes taking histories. But most top physicians agree that a thorough initial history requires at least fifteen minutes. This is only necessary at your first exam. At future checkups, your doctor needs only to ask you about your overall health and whether you developed any problems since your last exam. All of this information plus the findings of your exam become part of your medical chart.

Physical Exam

You may not feel medically deprived if you receive only routine Pap tests and contraceptive advice from your doctor. But when was the last time your doctor examined the rest of your body? If your doctor cannot meet your general health needs, find one who can. Make sure your physical exam includes:

> Urine test for possible urinary tract infection and diabetes.
> Blood test for possible anemia.
> Measurement of weight and height.
> Measurement of blood pressure (essential if you use the birth control pill).
> Examination of eyes, ears, nose, and throat.
> Palpation, or feeling of the neck, for glands or thyroid nodules.
> Listening to the lungs and heart with a stethoscope.
> Palpation of abdominal organs for tenderness, hernia, or an unusual mass.
> Checking of reflexes with a rubber hammer.
> Examination of your breasts sitting up and lying down. Your doctor should also instruct you in the method of breast self-examination. (See Chapter 20, Self-Examination.)
> Other tests as your health needs vary.

Pelvic Exam

No one really looks forward to this exam. In fact, some women actually hate it or are embarrassed by it. But that doesn't mean you should avoid it altogether. If you are over eighteen, have regular checkups. Unless you have an urgent problem, schedule your checkups between menstrual periods. While it is possible to have this exam done during the menstrual period, Pap tests are less accurate when mixed with menstrual blood. However, if your problem is one of constant bleeding or spotting, don't wait for it to stop. In addition, don't use douches, vaginal spermicides, or vaginal medications during the 24 hours before your exam, since these can also interfere with an accurate Pap test.

Your doctor starts off the exam by checking your external

genitals (vulva) for any irritation, infection, growth, or swellings. Next, your doctor inserts a stainless steel or plastic speculum into your vagina. (If it is cold, ask to have it warmed with water.) Once the speculum is in place, your doctor can check your vagina and cervix for any unusual discharge, infection, inflammation, or growths. At this point, a Pap test for the detection of abnormal cervical cells is taken. In this simple, quick, painless test your doctor collects some cells from your cervical canal and cervix. A medical laboratory determines whether the cells appear normal or abnormal and, if abnormal, to what degree. The final report is then sent to your doctor. The best thing about the Pap test is its ability to detect cervical dysplasia and very early cancer (also known as cancer *in situ*). These symptom-free conditions are nearly 100 percent curable if treated early.

Yet there is controversy about how often women should have a Pap test. The American Cancer Society and the American College of Obstetricians and Gynecologists continue to advocate the yearly Pap test. However, numerous research

Speculum exam with Pap test

speculum in place in vagina

cervix

collecting cells for the Pap test

studies have challenged the necessity of the yearly Pap. For example, one well-quoted Canadian study points out that women at "low-risk" for developing cervical conditions need only have a Pap once every three to five years providing the first two Pap tests are negative. But women at "high-risk" still need to continue having a Pap at least once a year. Until this issue is settled (if it ever is), ask your doctor how often you should have a pelvic exam with a Pap test.

The remainder of the exam is done without the speculum. After withdrawing the speculum, your doctor inserts one or two fingers into your vagina. By placing the other hand on your abdomen, your doctor can check your uterus, ovaries, and Fallopian tubes for any growths, tenderness, or other problems. Palpation of the uterus is not usually painful, but you may feel a twinge of pain when your doctor feels your ovaries. Your doctor completes the exam by inserting one finger into your vagina and one into your rectum to further check your reproductive organs for any problems. In addition, your rectum is felt for possible hemorrhoids, polyps, or other growths. If you find this a bit uncomfortable, try relaxing and taking deep breaths. The more relaxed you are

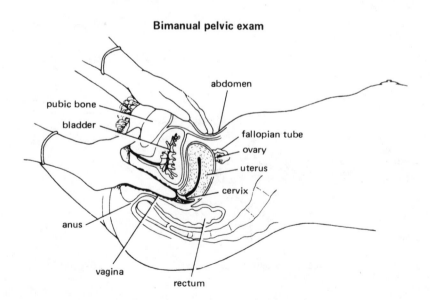

Bimanual pelvic exam

abdomen

pubic bone

bladder

fallopian tube

ovary

uterus

cervix

anus

vagina

rectum

during the exam, the easier it will be for both you and your doctor.

Your exam is over. Afterward, your doctor should tell you the findings of your exam, when to expect the results of your Pap test, and when to schedule your next health care check-up. If you want a method of birth control, compare the different methods and choose one with the help of your doctor.

If your exam uncovers some sort of problem, ask your doctor about:

- The medical diagnosis of your problem. (For example, the medical term "Trichomonas" is a lot more precise than vaginal infection.)
- The nature and prognosis of your problem. Make sure your doctor explains it in words you understand. For example, will it go away by itself without treatment, does it require only minor treatment, or is it life-threatening?
- The rationale for any recommended tests and treatment. (If your doctor recommends major surgery, ask about all alternative types of treatment open to you, and get a second surgical opinion about the necessity of surgery.)
- An explanation of any prescribed medication. How often to take it; when to take it (in the morning or evening, for example); how long to continue it; what side effects (if any) to expect; and whether to avoid certain foods or beverages while on the drug.
- When to schedule your next checkup and how long you will be under a doctor's care.
- Any other questions you feel are necessary to clearly understand the nature of your problem.

Most importantly, if you don't understand what your doctor is saying, say so.

☐ PATIENT RIGHTS

Some of the bigger news in health care today is being made by patients, not doctors. The issue is patient rights. People now want more facts from their doctors about their health and a bigger say in their treatment. Things were different until the mid-1960s — a time when doctors and their trade organization, the American Medical Association, had almost complete control over the medical profession. Since then, consumer groups have put great pressure on medical organizations and legislators to insure that doctors give their patients complete medical information. Already there have been several results. In 1973, the American Hospital Association adopted and distributed to its seven thousand member hospitals "A Patient's Bill of Rights" — the first formal statement spelling out how a patient should be treated in a hospital. It all adds up to better medical care and the chance for you to get more facts from your doctor during your hospital stay.

You now have the right to:

- Considerate and respectful care.
- Complete, current information concerning your diagnosis, treatment, and prognosis, in words you can understand; and to know the name of the doctor responsible for your care.
- Receive from your doctor whatever information you think is necessary to give your informed consent before the start of any medical procedure and/or treatment. Informed consent should explain the procedure and/or treatment, its risks, side effects, and alternative types of medical treatment that exist for you. (Informed consent may be verbal but is usually written; both forms are legally valid.) You also have the right to know who is responsible for your procedure and/or treatment.
- Refuse treatment to the extent permitted by law and to be informed of the medical consequences of your action.
- Every consideration of your privacy concerning your medical care program.
- Expect that all communications and records related to your care will be treated confidentially.
- Expect, within reason, your hospital to respond to your requests for services.
- Get information about any relationship between your

hospital and other health care and educational institutions, if it relates to your care; and to get information (including names) about any professional relationship among people who are treating you.

- Be advised if your hospital plans to engage in or perform human research or experimental studies that would affect your care or treatment; if so, you have the right to refuse to participate in any of these studies.
- Expect reasonable continuity of care.
- Examine and receive an explanation of your bill, regardless of how you plan to pay it.
- Know what hospital rules and regulations apply to your conduct as a patient.

Despite all this progress, there are problems. Many doctors still oppose the whole idea of patient rights. They feel that patients should leave everything up to their doctor and just follow instructions. Moreover, very few hospitals make it a policy to distribute copies of a Bill of Rights to their patients. Right now, only California, Massachusetts, Michigan, Minnesota, and New York legally require all hospitals to distribute a Bill of Rights to all patients.

Whether you deal with a doctor or hospital resistant to volunteering full information or ones that gladly make available every resource, learn your rights to help you get the medical information you want.

TABLE 1. Example of the Medical History

NAME _____

DATE OF BIRTH _____ AGE _____

OCCUPATION _____

What brings you here today? _____

_____

PAST HISTORY

Have you ever had:

	YES	NO
High blood pressure		
Heart or blood vessel disease		
Varicose veins		
Migraine or unusual headaches		
Anemia		
Sickle-cell disease		
Diabetes		
Cancer		
Hormonal disease		
Liver disease		
Kidney or bladder disease		
Gallbladder disease		
Asthma		
Epilepsy		
Allergies		
German measles		
Tuberculosis		
Gonorrhea or syphilis		
Reproductive organ problems		
Problems with drugs or alcohol		
Other problems		

PRESENT HEALTH

Do you currently have problems with:

	YES	NO
Headaches		
Eyes, ears, nose, throat		
Breathing		
Breasts		
Heart or circulation		
Bladder or kidneys		
Digestion		
Bowels		
Back		
Weight		
Sex life		
Reproductive organs		
Skin		
Hands or feet		
Emotional health		
Other problems		

SURGERY

Year	Operation

FAMILY HISTORY

Has any blood relative had:

	YES	NO	WHO
Cancer			
Diabetes			
High blood pressure			
Heart disease			
Hormonal disease			
Tuberculosis			
Other problems			

GENERAL

Do you smoke? no____ moderate____ heavy____

Do you drink alcohol? no____ moderate____ heavy____

What medications are you currently taking? ____

Are you allergic or sensitive to any drugs? ____

Do you examine your breasts monthly? ____

Any other health problems? ____

PREGNANCY HISTORY

Baby	Year	Months Pregnant	Type of Delivery	Complications
1.				
2.				
3.				
4.				
Others				

MENSTRUAL HISTORY

Are your periods normal? ____

Age at first period? ____

How often do you have periods? ____ days

Date last period began ____

Are your periods: regular ____ irregular ____ days

Length of periods ____

Usual flow: light ____ moderate ____ heavy ____

Do you have discomfort or pain before, during, or after your periods? ____

Discharge and/or bleeding between periods? ____

Your method of birth control (if any) ____

Any problems or side effects with your method of birth control? ____

Do you ever have pain during intercourse? ____

If postmenopausal, age and symptoms at menopause? ____

Do you have regular Pap tests? ____

Date of last Pap ____ Result ____

Any other menstrual problems? ____

2

MENSTRUAL CYCLE

Called by names as varied as *period, curse, monthlies, that time of the month, on the rag, the blues, the blahs, female problem,* and *flying the red flag,* the word menstruation is rarely used. Contrary to what some men and women believe, menstruation — despite its long list of derogatory nicknames — is a normal, natural, cyclic function. It is not — as some taboos, myths, and old wives' tales suggest — designed to rid the body of bad blood or various poisons. Menstruating women do not cause crops to blight, milk to sour, food to spoil, cake to fall, mayonnaise to curdle, and many other kitchen catastrophes to occur.

Even so, from the beginning of time menstruation inspired fear and awe. It magically set women apart from men in a mysterious way. Coming and going with regularity, it did not bring sickness or death. In many primitive societies women were excluded from daily activities for four to five days every month. They went instead to a menstrual hut some distance away from their village. There a menstruating woman might be "purified" or enjoy her solitude. Even until this century, women were advised to avoid bathing, swimming, or cold drinks. And right now women are still viewed as unreliable workers at that time of the month.

Fortunately, things are changing. We have come a long way from the myths about menstruation. Moreover, medical researchers continue to learn more about the normal menstrual cycle and the best way to treat its problems. Much of what is discussed in this chapter will help you understand and deal with common menstrual problems. As will be seen,

21

every woman has her own cycle. If you notice a significant change in your cycle, be sure to consult a doctor for evaluation of your symptoms, rather than using this chapter as a guide to self-diagnosis.

☐ PHYSIOLOGY OF THE MENSTRUAL CYCLE

Ask a woman what menstruation is and you may well get an incomplete answer. Though many women view it as only the monthly period, menstruation is much more than just periodic bleeding from the uterus. Your body actually operates in hormone-controlled cycles every month of your reproductive life, except during pregnancy. After menopause, menstrual cycles stop.

Briefly, the sequence of events in an average cycle follows this course. The first day of your cycle is the first day of menstrual bleeding, the shedding of the lining from your last cycle. During every cycle, when estrogen drops below a certain level, the pituitary (a small pea-sized gland at the base of the brain) releases a special hormone. This hormone, called follicle-stimulating hormone, stimulates one ovary to ripen a follicle and mature the egg it contains. When the egg matures, a large burst of another hormone from the pituitary (luteinizing hormone) helps release the egg from its follicle so that it can escape from the ovary. This process, called ovulation, occurs about 14 days before your period. This means that if you have a 28-day cycle, ovulation occurs on the 14th day; in a 34-day cycle it occurs on about the 20th day. As the egg escapes from the ovary, it is caught and drawn into one of the Fallopian tubes and starts its journey to the uterus, taking about five days to move three to five inches. As the egg starts to travel down the tube, the follicle that produced the egg acquires a new name, corpus luteum. The corpus luteum produces the hormones progesterone and estrogen, which prepare the lining of the uterus for possible pregnancy.

If your partner's sperm are present in your tubes and conditions are favorable, one sperm unites with your egg (Conception, see Chapter 6). Over the next several days the fertilized egg travels down the tube to the uterus where it implants itself in the already-prepared lining of the uterus. Under the combined influence of estrogen and progesterone, the lining of the uterus has been built up to receive the egg, hold it in place, and sustain it through pregnancy. The uterus grows thick and spongy, and stores up blood and other nutrients. After the fertilized egg implants itself in the uterus, the fetus develops in the uterus during the nine months of pregnancy.

If, however, your egg is not fertilized, it disintegrates before getting to your uterus. Since pregnancy did not occur in that cycle, the lining of the uterus (endometrium) and the stored-up blood are no longer needed. For this reason, the top layers of the endometrium are shed away from the uterus. This flow — called menstrual flow, *menses*, or menstruation — usually dark red blood with bits of mucus and fragments of the endometrium, passes out of the uterus, through the cervix and vagina, and out of the body. Then a new menstrual cycle begins.

The first menstrual period (menarche) occurs several years after puberty, usually between the ages of 11 and 14. Having a first period as early as age nine or as late as 16 can happen and is not necessarily abnormal. And, according to statistics, the average age has been getting younger and younger. For example, the average age of menarche 100 years ago in the United States was 14. Now it is 12½ years of age. Girls who have their first period before age nine or who do not have their first period by 18 should receive medical consultation. This is because hormonal disorders as well as other problems can be responsible for either an early or late menarche. Menstrual periods continue until age 45 to 55, at which time the ovaries cease their function and menstrual periods permanently stop. (See Chapter 21, Menopause.)

For the first few years after menarche and shortly before menopause, the menstrual cycles are often irregular in length and amount of flow. This is because they are "anovulatory" cycles; that is, they occur without ovulation. Even though hormones cause the lining of the uterus to shed, producing menstrual flow, no egg erupts from the ovaries. This means that some (but certainly not all) young teenagers and menopausal women are not fertile. (So you still need to use some method of birth control.) Once a woman starts to ovulate — anywhere from three months to three to four years after the first period — menstrual periods become regular and fertility begins.

The amount and length of flow varies widely from woman to woman, and, for that matter, may change throughout a woman's life. Counting day one as the first day of bleeding, most women have cycles that are 24 to 34 days long, with an average of 28 days. Deviations of six or seven days every so often are not abnormal. The amount of blood lost during a period varies from one to six ounces with an average of two ounces. Usually the flow is greater on the first two days, followed by a gradual tapering off. Though bleeding can vary from one to eight days, most women flow for about five days.

□ **PAIN AT OVULATION**

Pain with ovulation (*Mittelschmerz*) is fairly common. Occurring at midcycle during ovulation, symptoms consist of cramping pains on one or both sides of the lower abdomen. These cramps may be coupled with some vaginal discharge, sometimes slight bleeding. Most women with *Mittelschmerz* have only transient twinges of pain for less than a day. But, occasionally, the symptoms of ovulation are painful enough to mimic appendicitis or pregnancy outside the uterus (ectopic pregnancy), in which case you should call a doctor promptly.

If you have severe midcycle pain and/or bleeding, consult a doctor for advice and evaluation of your symptoms. And — since pain from other abdominal organs can be confused with ovulatory pain — don't use this pain phenomenon either as proof of ovulation or as a signal to abstain from intercourse for birth control.

☐ PREMENSTRUAL TENSION

Three to seven days before their periods — occasionally as long as 10 to 14 days — most women experience symptoms that alert them of their approaching period. Symptoms may include one or more of the following: general feelings of depression, fatigue, irritability, lack of concentration; small outbreaks of acne; headache and backache; nausea, constipation, or diarrhea; tight feelings in the pelvic area and legs; breast tenderness and swelling; and a bloated and puffy feeling in the abdomen. Some women temporarily gain several pounds of weight because of fluid retention. Most women have only a few mild symptoms, and, for this reason, are able to carry out their normal activities without consulting a doctor for treatment. When, however, symptoms are severe enough to disrupt normal activities, they constitute a syndrome known as *premenstrual tension*. In addition to the above symptoms (which may or may not be present) women with premenstrual tension show noticeable personality changes that end abruptly with the start of the period. Changes begin gradually with signs of anxiety, depression, irritability, and progress to restlessness, emotional outbursts, anger, and a host of other related mood changes.

What actually causes symptoms before the period is not always clear. Frequently the symptoms are associated with the body's ability to retain greater amounts of salt and water just before menstrual flow starts. Most doctors attribute this biological activity to a temporary imbalance between estrogen and progesterone. Whether symptoms are brought about by too much estrogen, too little progesterone, or from some other hormonal factor, nobody knows for sure. Sometimes these physical changes in addition to emotional, social, and personal problems can play a role in causing symptoms. If your symptoms are mild, the simple act of restricting your salt intake seven to ten days before your period can be quite helpful. Such foods as ham, bacon, sausage, lunch meat, hot dogs, potato chips, nuts, and Chinese and Mexican cooking are especially high in salt.

If you have severe symptoms that begin a week or more

before your period, consult a doctor. To control the symptoms related to fluid retention, doctors often prescribe a diet low in salt during the premenstrual week coupled with diuretics. This prescription drug stimulates the kidneys to eliminate excess fluids. Less frequently — when diuretics do not relieve all the symptoms — doctors prescribe a mild tranquilizer or hormone therapy, such as the birth control pill.

☐ LUMPY BREASTS

About a week before their periods, most women experience breast fullness and tenderness, caused by fluid retention and altered hormone levels. A normal reaction to the approaching period, it is part and parcel of other premenstrual symptoms.

During the reproductive years, repeated episodes of monthly breast changes may lead to lumpy breasts (fibrocystic disease). It usually makes its appearance during the thirties and is very common in the forties. Fibrocystic disease can appear in a variety of forms: both breasts may be only painful and tender; breasts may feel fuller, heavier, and a bit lumpy; or one or more cysts — small or large — may be felt. Women with fibrocystic disease often notice breast changes throughout their menstrual cycle. Generally, symptoms are worst before the menstrual period and then subside or disappear after the period. Likewise, cysts may come and go with the period, remain stable, or disappear completely from time to time. Fibrocystic disease is largely a self-limited disease. It slowly disappears after the menopause but may reappear in women using estrogen replacement therapy.

For women bothered by breast fullness and tenderness, wearing a good uplift bra during the week before the period is usually all that is needed. If, according to your doctor, you have fibrocystic disease, your symptoms can be relieved. (See Chapter 20, Common Benign Breast Diseases.) To ease pain, restriction of salt and fluids along with wearing a good bra may be all that is necessary. To rid the breasts of excess fluids, diuretics as well as hormones can provide relief. If you have a particularly painful cyst, your doctor may drain fluid from it (needle aspiration). Often, the cyst does not come back and relief is permanent. If it persists or returns one to two months later, consult your doctor for further evaluation. Though most breast lumps are benign breast disease — and not breast cancer — it is essential that your doctor determine the nature of any type of breast lump.

Whether you have fibrocystic disease or not, you can help yourself and your doctor if you practice monthly breast self-examination. While examining your breasts, pay attention to the changes that occur in your breasts with each menstrual cycle. Only by becoming familiar with your breasts under normal conditions, will you recognize something different that your doctor should check. (See Chapter 20, Self-Examination, for when and how to examine your breasts.)

☐ **PAINFUL PERIODS**

Painful or uncomfortable periods (*dysmenorrhea*) are the most common problem associated with the menstrual cycle. At some time in their lives, most women experience painful periods; that is, cramps or constant pain in the lower abdomen. Other symptoms may also include pain in the thighs, backache, headache (sometimes migraine), nausea, vomiting, and a general overall feeling of discomfort.

Symptoms vary from mild to severe and are generally worst on the first day of menstrual flow. Milder symptoms may also occur one to two days before and after the first day. If symptoms are mild, there is no cause for alarm. In fact, many women have only mildly uncomfortable periods and are able to continue their activities with the help of a few aspirin. Other women are disabled to the point of being bedridden for a day or two each period. If your symptoms are severe every month, be sure to consult a doctor for advice and treatment.

The causes of painful periods vary widely. *Primary dysmen-*

orrhea, the commonest kind, is painful periods without any underlying problem. While little is known about the cause of primary dysmenorrhea, one currently well-regarded theory states that a high level of prostaglandins in the menstrual flow may cause abdominal cramps. Prostaglandins, fat-like substances manufactured by the lining of the uterus and other organs, resemble hormones. Symptoms of primary dysmenorrhea usually begin in the late teens, two or three years after the first menstrual period (after ovulation starts). They often last for the next few years or, in a mild form, for the rest of a woman's menstruating years. Frequently the problem fades by itself after childbirth — for reasons that are not clear.

Aspirin and a routine of daily exercises can often provide relief of mild to moderate cramps. Until recently it was thought that the effectiveness of aspirin was due only to its pain-relieving characteristics. It is now known that aspirin actually blocks the production of prostaglandins, which helps explain why aspirin work so well. Two aspirin every four hours is usually sufficient for an average-sized woman. For women who cannot tolerate aspirin, one of the over-the-counter pain medications may be helpful. Additionally, a warm tub, heating pad against the abdomen, or a small amount of liquor also may bring relief. Interestingly, having an orgasm is credited with relieving cramps, probably because this dilates the pelvic blood vessels.

If you have tried all of these remedies without success, or your symptoms are severe, contact a doctor. Ideally, you should try to get relief with as little medication as possible. Generally, doctors first prescribe a mild pain killer or a medication containing codeine. The regular use of codeine — a narcotic that may cause potential addiction — has obvious disadvantages. If your symptoms persist after several months of trying pain medications, your doctor may prescribe the birth control pill for a trial period of two to three months. By stopping ovulation the Pill diminishes activity within the uterus, where most pains originate. If your periods remain painful despite the Pill, further medical evaluation is necessary to determine the cause of your painful menstrual periods.

Some women develop *secondary dysmenorrhea*, which generally starts in the late twenties or early thirties after years of relatively pain-free periods. Unlike primary dysmenorrhea, it is secondary to a specific problem. Common causes are endometriosis, fibroids, pelvic inflammatory disease, or endometrial polyps. (See Chapter 5.) Only after a doctor determines the cause of your symptoms during a complete gynecologic checkup can you receive treatment.

Another possible cause of secondary dysmenorrhea is the intrauterine device (IUD). In some women — especially those who have never been pregnant — the IUD may cause menstrual cramps and bleeding. (See Chapter 8, Side Effects.) Since IUDs come in different shapes and sizes, replacement with a different one may solve the problem. In fact, medicated IUDs, such as the Progestasert, apparently have fewer uncomfortable side effects. If trying a new IUD doesn't work, consider choosing another method of birth control.

☐ HEAVY PERIODS

Excessive bleeding — during either a normal or long menstrual period — may occur from time to time. Yet it happens most frequently at the beginning and toward the end of reproductive life — in teenagers and premenopausal women over 40. If you develop *any* type of bleeding after your menopause (defined as 12 months after your last period), see a doctor promptly. While it is difficult to determine how much is too much, if you have to use more feminine napkins or tampons compared with your normal periods, or notice large clots in your menstrual flow, consult a doctor.

Heavy periods are often due to a shift in hormone levels, such as failure to ovulate every cycle. Less frequently the cause may be one of several endocrine disorders; pelvic inflammatory disease; endometriosis; fibroids; cancer; or even emotional factors. If you develop heavy periods, consult a doctor for evaluation of your symptoms. Only after a doctor determines the cause of your symptoms during a complete medical checkup can you receive treatment for this problem.

☐ BLEEDING BETWEEN PERIODS

Light bleeding or spotting for a day or so between periods may or may not signal trouble. This symptom may have normal causes such as shifting hormone levels at or near the time of ovulation, or just before or after the menstrual period. On the other hand, if you have heavy bleeding between periods, the problem may involve such causes as: endocrine disorders; pelvic inflammatory disease; endometriosis; fibroids; polyps; or cancer.

Whether you have light or heavy bleeding between your periods, consult a doctor, who may want to do a biopsy or D and C. (See Chapter 18.) Only after a doctor determines the cause of the abnormal bleeding can you receive treatment.

☐ IRREGULAR AND MISSED PERIODS

Irregular periods — arriving earlier or later than usual — and missed periods may be the result of emotional as well as physical factors. For example, going away to school or college, a change in residence, medications such as tranquilizers and the birth control pill, or a death in the family can bring about irregular or missed periods. Similarly, physical factors such as any long-standing chronic illness, the flu, or even crash diets can upset normal periods in some women. Though these symptoms occur from time to time in all women, irregular and missed periods are much more common at the beginning and end of reproductive life — when the hormone system is least predictable.

Amenorrhea, complete lack of menstrual periods, can have

any number of causes. *Primary amenorrhea* means failure to menstruate by about age 16. Often an endocrine problem, such as an ovarian disorder, is at fault. Less frequently such causes as a completely closed or "imperforate" hymen, underdevelopment of the reproductive system, underlying disease, or emotional factors are responsible. *Secondary amenorrhea*, on the other hand, is the absence of menstruation for longer than three periods in already menstruating women. Causes of secondary amenorrhea may include: pregnancy; breast-feeding and the post-partum period; menopause; endocrine problems; underlying disease; emotional factors; extreme weight loss; or long-term use of tranquilizers or the birth control pill.

If you have primary or secondary amenorrhea, consult a doctor for evaluation of your symptoms. Only after a doctor determines the cause of your amenorrhea during a complete medical checkup can you receive treatment.

□ **MENSTRUAL HEALTH**

Menstrual periods require no special activity on your part, except for sanitary precautions. Whether you choose to use one of the more common methods of absorbing menstrual flow, such as tampons or feminine napkins, is a matter of personal choice. Many women enjoy the convenience of tampons. Being a virgin should not stop you from using tampons, since most women have hymens able to accommodate at least a small tampon. If you are new at using tampons, each box has an insert with easy-to-follow instructions.

Menstrual or *period extraction* is another way to control menstrual periods. Practiced by self-help feminist groups, this method aims at avoiding the discomfort or inconvenience of a monthly period. Just before the period is due, a woman or one of her friends inserts a special tube into the uterus. This tube, attached to a source of suction, gently and rapidly sucks out the lining of the uterus normally shed during the menstrual period. By eliminating belts, pads, pins, tampons, and menstrual discomfort, menstrual extraction gives a woman complete control of her body. But right now the long-term safety of using this method every month is unknown.

Feminine deodorant sprays to mask menstrual odors are unnecessary and may actually do more harm than good. In fact, side effects such as itching and burning of the vulva, vagina, and the sex partner's penis now prohibit their use on tampons, feminine napkins, or before sexual intercourse. All that is really needed for an odor-free genital area is soap and water.

Douching after your period (or at any time during the month) is okay. If you must douche, limit it to once or twice a week. Though there are many commercial douches available, two tablespoons of white vinegar in a quart of warm water is just as good and a lot cheaper. Douching actually is unnecessary and many doctors dispute its usefulness. This is because the vagina cleanses itself through drainage and bacterial action. Also, too frequent and improper douching with strong solutions can actually alter the vagina's natural protective mechanisms.

Contrary to what some women believe, you can and should continue your normal activities — such as baths, showers, exercise, fresh air, enough rest and sleep, personal hygiene, a well-balanced diet, and socializing — during your menstrual period. Moreover, physical activities (even swimming) during the period are okay. Recent medical studies show that women who are physically active as a matter of routine have fewer menstrual problems, including headaches, fatigue, and cramps. These studies also show that exercise — more than anything else — helps prevent and relieve menstrual cramps by increasing blood circulation and releasing muscle tensions. (In the last three Olympics women won gold medals and established new world records during every phase of the menstrual cycle.)

Although any daily exercise routine will help, the best exercises are bending and stretching to work the muscles in the abdomen and lower back. Exercise programs — done at home out of a book or as part of a class under trained supervision — vary considerably. For this reason, consult a doctor or an exercise specialist about what is best for you. If exercises are going to help, you won't notice relief for several months.

Sexual activity during your menstrual period is a matter of choice between you and your partner. What's more, it is medically harmless. Some men and women—for personal or religious reasons—prefer not to have intercourse during a woman's period. They find it offensive and psychologically difficult. The idea that a woman is unclean or untouchable during her period is not true, so do what you prefer. It turns out, though, that some women experience increased sexual drive and sensitivity during their menstrual period.

3

SEXUALITY

Remember the days when no one talked openly about sex? Well, things have changed. We now live in a much freer, more permissible age. As a result of this new sexual freedom, women now share their feelings about sexuality at women's groups, in neighborhood backyards, at PTA meetings, as well as other types of social gatherings. Moreover, never before have there been so many books on sex. Books on sex techniques, self-help sex therapy, and sexuality are selling by the million. As part of this changing climate, women have become increasingly aware of their own sexuality and what it means in terms of *total* self-expression. What's more, women now expect more from their sexual relationships. And — with changing cultural attitudes toward bisexuality and homosexuality — more women are now exploring different sexual lifestyles.

This chapter does not have all the answers on how to have a perfect sex life or explore all the dimensions of sexuality. Instead, it covers a range of topics from sexual anatomy and intercourse to sex problems and therapy. Let's take a look at the basics.

☐ A WOMAN'S REPRODUCTIVE ORGANS

Knowing your sexual and reproductive anatomy and physiology is not as difficult as it sounds. If you never really examined yourself, get a hand mirror, a room with good light, and proceed. Many women find squatting on the floor or sitting on the edge of a chair a good position. If you are uncomfortable doing this, spend a few seconds the first time. Later on, look for a while longer.

Outer Organs

First, you will immediately see a triangular area covered with hair. It starts from a soft pad of fatty tissue (*mons*); press against this pad and find your underlying pubic bone. Notice that the area covered with pubic hair divides and continues on either side for three to four inches. These fatty folds of flesh or outer larger lips are called the *labia majora*. They cushion the inner area and keep it moist. Separating the larger lips, you can clearly see the inner smaller lips (*labia minora*). They are hairless and far more sensitive than the larger ones. During sexual stimulation, they darken and become firm.

Look more closely and you will see the inner lips joining to form a soft fold of skin or *hood* over the clitoris. Though

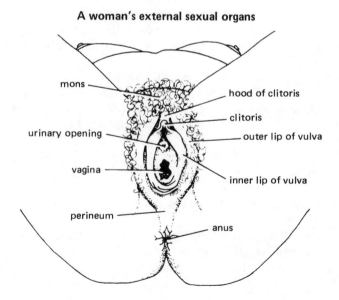

A woman's external sexual organs

mons
hood of clitoris
clitoris
urinary opening
outer lip of vulva
vagina
inner lip of vulva
perineum
anus

most of the *clitoris* is actually hidden under this fold of skin, you can see its tip or *glans* which looks like the size of a pink pencil eraser. The clitoris varies in size from woman to woman but is usually one-sixth to one-half inch long. During sexual excitement, it swells with blood and becomes firm and erect — nearly doubling in size. As for its function, the clitoris is the source of sexual sensation and orgasm.

The opening to the bladder (*urethra*) lies just below the clitoris. Finding it can be difficult, since it looks like a small dot or slit. This thin tube — only about an inch and a half long — carries urine from the bladder to outside the body.

Beneath the urethra is the *hymen* or its remnants if you have had sexual intercourse. Sometimes called the maidenhead or cherry, the hymen is a thin membrane. Coming in an array of sizes and shapes, it partially blocks the entrance to the vagina. Most hymens can fit the passage of a finger or tampon; rarely are they completely closed or "imperforate." (Since closed hymens also trap menstrual periods in the vagina, the lack of menstrual periods in well-developed girls usually leads to early medical diagnosis and correction of this problem.) During first intercourse, this opening — with a little bit of tearing and slight bleeding — gets broken by the erect penis. Under ordinary circumstances, this is an untraumatic event. The hymen further gets destroyed during delivery of the first baby. Afterward, there are only a few of its remains. (These tattered remains are of no importance, but some women may mistake them for small growths.) An intact hymen — generally regarded as a sign of virginity — can be broken by things other than intercourse. Strenuous exercise — such as horseback riding — can sometimes result in rupture, as well as masturbation with fingers in the vagina.

So far you have identified your outer organs or the various parts of your *vulva*. Let's proceed to the inner organs.

Inner Organs

If you have never examined your vagina, insert a finger or two into it. If you need lubrication, baby oil, K-Y jelly, or cold cream will do. Sweep your fingers around the walls and feel how stretchable they are. Notice if your walls are dry or wet. (This varies depending on whether you are in your reproductive years and, if so, where you are in your menstrual cycle.) Try to tighten your vagina around your finger. (Imagine you are trying to stop urinating.) You are now contracting your *pelvic floor muscles.* If these muscles are weak, you may have trouble having orgasm, controlling your urine (causes stress incontinence), or your pelvic organs (causes prolapse of the bladder or uterus, for example).

Slide your middle finger to the top of your vagina and notice the far end seems to be closed. This means it is impossible for tampons, diaphragms, and the like to get lost up there. Continue to explore and you will find your *cervix* or base of the uterus. One to two inches across, it feels about as firm as the end of your nose. Notice the small dimple in the center. It is the opening of the cervix or *cervical os.*

At this point, you will not be able to feel the rest of your inner reproductive organs. Beyond the cervix lies the main body of the *uterus.* The uterus does not lie in a direct straight line with the vagina. Instead, it normally tips a little forward (anteverted). In about one out of five women, the uterus tilts back (retroverted). Rarely does a retroverted uterus cause any problems.

The nonpregnant uterus is about the size and shape of an upside down pear. It is so stretchable that during pregnancy it can blow up bigger than a king-size watermelon. Afterward, it reverts to its former size. The uterus plays many roles: it is responsible for menstruation; helping transport sperm; holding the fertilized egg; and developing the fetus through the nine months of pregnancy.

The two reproductive glands, the *ovaries,* are located on either side of the upper uterus. During the menstruating years, the ovaries are about the size of two unshelled almonds. After the menopause, they shrink. Ovaries have two primary functions: to produce an egg every menstrual cycle and secrete the female sex hormones, estrogen and progesterone. These hormones help maintain female sex characteristics (such as firm breasts and lubricated vaginal tissues), regulate the menstrual cycle, and support pregnancy.

A woman's pelvic organs

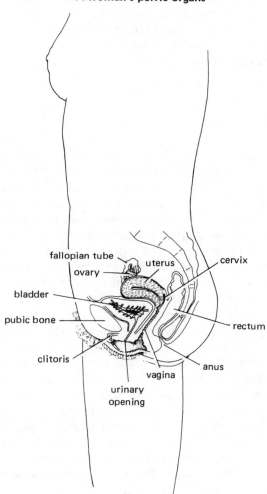

Extending about four inches out of either side of the uterus are the *Fallopian tubes*, one serving each ovary. Each tube wraps part way around its ovary, but is not attached to it. During ovulation, the tentacle-like ends of the tubes (*fimbriae*) sweep across the entire surface of the ovaries to pick up the egg when it arrives. If an egg is not fertilized by a sperm in the Fallopian tube within 24 hours or so, it disintegrates. If it gets fertilized, the Fallopian tube maintains the fertilized egg while it makes its five to six day journey to the lining of the uterus.

☐ SEXUAL INTERCOURSE

If you think there is any right, or expected, or standard way to relate sexually, you are wrong. Stereotyped sex — filling two to three ritualized minutes at night, for example — is scarcely the way to get or give much pleasure. Many couples develop hang-ups about the man-on-top position, having orgasms together, having intercourse so many times a week, and so on. Rather than lock yourself into a conventional sex life, realize there are many different ways of getting and giving sexual pleasure. In fact, being spontaneous — free to do what you want — is really best.

It all starts off with getting turned on, or foreplay. Whether this entails caressing each other's bodies and genitals, kissing, oral-genital stimulation, or any other sort of affectionate expression, doesn't matter. What is important here is spontaneity and mutual stimulation. No one should take a passive role during this stage or any other stage of sex. You can increase your own pleasure and your partner's by actively engaging in foreplay. If — like most women — you need manual stimulation of your clitoris to get aroused, include it as an active part of foreplay. How long to spend on foreplay is up to you. Some couples find a few minutes adequate, while others enjoy a half hour or more.

Apart from being psychologically stimulating, foreplay prepares both you and your partner for intercourse. As sexual tensions mount, your vagina normally becomes very wet and lubricated and your partner gets an erection. (If your vagina tends to stay dry, use a lubricant such as K-Y jelly before sex to lubricate your vagina and area around your clitoris.) When you are sufficiently aroused, take your partner's penis into your vagina. Over time, you will know when you are ready to begin intercourse.

There is no proper, normal position-to-end-all-positions for intercourse. (If you are looking for variety, see Readings and Resources.) Though face-to-face positions do seem to be most popular, chances are your favorite position will change from time to time with mood and experience. Though many couples find the man-on-top as the most acceptable position, it is not uncommon for the woman to take the uppermost position. In one example of the "female superior" position, the woman crouches over her partner in a sitting position, her knees on either side of his body, and slides back and forth on his penis. The advantage here is that you can caress and look at each other at the same time. For many women, this is the easiest and sometimes the only way to achieve orgasm with intercourse. It is also a good position for manual stimulation of the clitoris. This is especially important for women who need this kind of stimulation to reach orgasm.

Once you are in position, begin moving rhythmically together. If you are not aroused enough but your partner is highly aroused, move your pelvis slowly — rather than quickly — against his. In addition to up-and-down movements, add some variety such as circular motions. With experience, you will learn how to arouse and excite each other.

Ideally, if you both pace yourself, you can reach orgasm together or within minutes of each other. More often than not, this is the exception rather than the rule. In fact, less than half of all women have an orgasm during intercourse. But recent studies suggest if you include manual clitoral stimulation during foreplay *and* intercourse, it is much easier to have an orgasm during intercourse. Otherwise — if the clitoris gets only indirect stimulation during vaginal intercourse from its hood sliding back and forth over it — it is more difficult to have an orgasm.

According to researchers, sex is more than just foreplay and orgasm. Close investigations show it is actually a sequence of four phases which — for both men and women — make up the "sexual response cycle." This cycle follows the same course whether you reach orgasm through sexual intercourse, masturbation, or some other activity.

The first phase of the sexual response cycle is the *excitement phase*, which in the man produces an erection and in the woman vaginal lubrication and swelling of all the sex organs. But this phase is not limited to the sex organs. It is a total body response: nipples become erect and the breasts larger; chest and neck become flushed; heart rate increases; breathing becomes faster and deeper; body muscles begin to tighten, especially in the genitals. The second phase, the *plateau phase*, is basically a continual buildup of all the changes in the excitement phase.

As tension builds to a peak, orgasm then occurs. Contrary to what you may have heard or read, all orgasms are not the same. Not only do they vary from woman to woman, but even the same woman can have different experiences with orgasm. Sometimes it may be a very mild experience, like a ripple; or a warm, glowing experience; or an almost seizure-like, tension releasing experience; or an extremely intense experience with a momentary loss of awareness. And some women can have several orgasms in a row if continually stimulated. (What is important is not how many you have, but what satisfies you.) The man's orgasm is very much like the woman's, except that it features an ejaculation of semen. This fluid, which contains sperm, is ejected from the penis in three to seven spurts. After orgasm, during the *resolution phase*, both men and women experience profound relaxation throughout their bodies. For those who reach the plateau stage but not orgasm, this phase can be uncomfortable; that is, it can take over an hour to feel relaxed again.

Over the years there has been a lot of controversy over the merits of vaginal versus clitoral orgasm. The psychoanalyst Sigmund Freud sparked it off in the 1930s by insisting there are two distinct kinds of orgasms. The clitoral type, he said, was usually achieved through masturbation, making it an immature, childish form of sexual gratification. For the mature, well-adjusted woman, he declared, orgasm originates in the vagina during intercourse and — for this reason — is more intense and fulfilling. Until recently, these observations went largely unquestioned.

Sex researchers have now observed hundreds of couples and single individuals engaging in nearly every sort of sexual activity. Evidence shows there is no such thing as vaginal or clitoral orgasms. It is all a myth. The clitoris is unquestionably the source of sexual sensation and orgasm. But it can be stimulated by sexual intercourse as well as by manual stimulation. Thus no type of orgasm is more real or more right than any other. Both are simply orgasms.

In addition to sexual intercourse, there are other ways of getting and giving sexual pleasure. For example, you can mutually stroke or lick each others genitals to orgasm. Whether you do or don't have oral sex is up to you, but for many couples it is one of the most pleasurable and exciting forms of sexual activity. And there is anal sex — a highly erotic form of stimulation for some couples. If you have anal sex, be gentle and careful. The anus is not as elastic as the vagina, so use a lubricant such as K-Y jelly on your partner's penis. (Saliva is not enough.) Since anal bacteria can cause vaginal infections, make sure your partner's penis gets washed if you want it in your vagina after it has been in your anus.

Judging from the number of popular books on the subject, there are endless ways to excite each other sexually. (See Readings and Resources.) The pleasures of sex include a wide range of feelings and experiences, so explore and find out what satisfies you the most.

□ **MASTURBATION**

Despite strong cultural and religious biases against it, masturbation or self-stimulation is a common and healthy way of obtaining sexual pleasure. It is important to free yourself of any notions you may have that it is unhealthy, immoral, or immature. It is a source of pleasure to be learned and enjoyed for its own sake. In fact, there are enough surveys to show that most women — whether married, single, sexually deprived, or enjoying an active sex life — have masturbated. These studies also show that masturbation brings the average woman to a faster, more intense orgasm than any other type of sexual stimulation. What's more, sex therapists advise masturbation for women having trouble reaching orgasm, to teach women about their bodies, promote satisfying orgasms, express one's full sexual potential, learn about multiple orgasms, and survive sexually without a partner. To most women, however, masturbation will never replace sexual intercourse with a partner. It is just not as much fun.

There are many ways to masturbate. It is true that most women masturbate by rubbing their fingers around and over their clitoris. But, there are other ways such as using a pillow instead of your hands or having sexual fantasies while you masturbate. Using a vibrator is still another way. Vibrators, which cause intense, dependable stimulation, are also used in sex therapy to teach women how to reach orgasm.

☐ SEXUAL PROBLEMS

If you have ever had a sexual problem—such as not being satisfied, or never coming to a climax, or finding sex boring and routine—realize you are not alone. At one time or an-another, one-half of all couples have some kind of problem with sex. Here are some of the more common ones women experience:

Lack of Orgasm

Remember the word frigid—*any* lack of sexual interest or response in women? In place of this imprecise, cruel, catch-all term, doctors now use more accurate labels for the various forms of this problem. The new terms are based on whether —and under what circumstances—a woman achieves orgasm. Women with *primary orgasmic dysfunction* never experience orgasm, except—on rare occasion—in dreams. This problem almost always has emotional causes, making any kind of orgasm, even with masturbation, very difficult. Women with *secondary orgasmic dysfunction* experience orgasm in one situation but not in another—for example, with masturbation but not during sexual intercourse.

The causes of this problem, which affects nearly half of all women, are many. For instance, guilt about sex is a common one. An overprotective or strict religious upbringing can (and frequently does) produce women unable to experience sexual pleasure. On the other hand, you may have no qualms whatever about sex, but certain everyday situations can and do arise. Here are some common ones: depression, stress, and fatigue; preoccupation with other things; overly aggressive or passive sexual partner; lack of trust or commitment in a relationship; anxiously trying to please your partner more than yourself; afraid to ask for what stimulates you (good sex doesn't come naturally); afraid to say you just don't feel like having sex at that moment. Less commonly, some medical problems and the use or overuse of certain drugs or alcohol can also affect orgasm. Not uncommonly -- when the romance suddenly evaporates in a relationship—many women have difficulty achieving orgasm. Or maybe your partner has a sexual problem which is contributing to your problem. Sex studies show that about one-half of all women who never reach orgasm have partners with some sort of problem, such as premature ejaculation.

Not having an orgasm every time you have sex is not abnormal. If you have never had an orgasm or only have them in one situation but not in another, see the next section on Sex Therapy.

Low Interest in Sex

Every woman's interest in sex varies from time to time. For example, just as there are days in the menstrual cycle when women get highly interested in sex, there are also days when almost no amount of stimulation is exciting. Or maybe you have noticed there are times when your interest in sex is really low for weeks or even months. For instance, periods of intense work or study, depression and fatigue, relationship problems, times of important life change, and the post-partum period commonly affect sexual interest and response. Less commonly, some medical problems and the use or overuse of certain drugs or alcohol can also interfere with sexual interest and response. Being uninterested in sex for short periods of time is normal. If this continues to be a problem for you, see the next section on Sex Therapy.

Painful Intercourse

Dyspareunia or painful intercourse comes from the Greek word meaning "bad or difficult mating." In some women, the word is an apt one, since the pain may actually be a defense against a sexual situation they can't handle or wish to avoid. At other times, anxiety or guilt about sex may be the culprit. But painful intercourse can have any number of physical causes, and just about all women have it from time to time.

Insufficient vaginal lubrication is one of the most common causes of painful intercourse. Normally the walls of the vagina become wet and sweaty during foreplay. But when you let your partner's penis in too soon, or if you are anxious about sex, or if your partner uses a condom, you may need to add lubrication. Give your vagina time to get wet. If you still feel dry, use saliva, lubricating jelly (such as K-Y jelly), or vaginal spermicide. (Don't use petroleum jelly to lubricate a condom since it will destroy the rubber.) The menopause and low-dose birth control pills can also affect vaginal lubrication. If lubricating jelly doesn't help, see a doctor for treatment.

Local vaginal infection and irritation is another common cause of painful intercourse. Sexually-transmitted infections, as well as allergic reactions to feminine deodorant sprays, vaginal spermicides, and rubber (from a condom or diaphragm), can cause stingy, itchy intercourse. If you develop one of the sexually-transmitted infections in Chapter 4, see a doctor for treatment. Otherwise, stop using your feminine deodorant spray; switch your brand of vaginal spermicide; have your partner use a skin rather than rubber condom; or see a doctor about a plastic diaphragm.

Pain from an *overly snug vaginal opening* is not always limited to virgins or women with infrequent sexual experience. It can also occur in postmenopausal women because of vaginal changes. In addition, the stitches after vaginal delivery can temporarily tighten the vaginal opening. See a doctor if this continues to be a problem for you.

Pain deep inside the vagina or pelvis has any number of causes. Endometriosis (tissue from the endometrium growing outside the uterus) is one of the most notable examples. (See Chapter 5.) This creates a sharp, stabbing pain during deep penile thrusting, and it can truly make intercourse unbearable. Other causes may include: retroverted uterus; pelvic inflammatory disease; ovarian cyst; cancer of the reproductive system; extensive surgery; or radiation therapy for pelvic cancer. If you develop this symptom, see a doctor for medical diagnosis and treatment. Also, trying sexual positions not involving deep penile thrusting can sometimes bring relief.

Painful penetration or vaginismus — the least common sex problem — is even more restricting than painful intercourse. Not only is intercourse extremely painful, it is often impossible. This is because the muscles surrounding the lower vagina tighten and contract spastically. The problem itself is really a way of saying "no" to sex without actually saying the word. For some women, certain sexual situations can bring this about: for example, situations they can't handle or don't want to be in. For others, it can be the result of rape or even guilt about sex. If you develop this problem, see the next section on Sex Therapy.

□ SEX THERAPY

If you are troubled sexually, first go to your doctor to see if there is some physical reason for your problem, such as a local vaginal infection. If your exam is normal and the doctor feels that your problem can be helped by sex therapy, ask for a referral to a sex therapist. There are a lot of people calling themselves sex therapists who have little or no training in treating sexual problems. The important thing is to contact a sex therapist *fully* qualified to treat sex problems. So first contact your own doctor or clinic rather than using the Yellow Pages or a newspaper. If that doesn't work, call your nearest medical school or hospital affiliated with a medical school and ask for their human sexuality program. You can also contact the Eastern Association for Sex Therapists or the American Association of Sex Educators, Counselors, and Educators for a list of sex therapists and sex clinics throughout the country. (See Readings and Resources.)

There are several types of sex therapy, but sex therapy is not the answer for everyone. In fact, it is only helpful for about 50 percent of all people who go for help. (If you are reluctant to go for help, you might first want to try one of the self-help books listed in Readings and Resources.) Therapists get the best results in curing orgasm problems such as inability to reach orgasm in women and premature ejaculation in men. The cure rate here is nearly 90 percent. Over half of all people with excitement problems — such as insufficient vaginal lubrication and painful penetration in women and lack of erection in men — can be helped. Good sex therapy for these kinds of problems is usually two-fold. It includes a series of step-by-step exercises that both you *and* your partner do at home integrated with psychotherapy at the clinic. Often this type of treatment is quick and effective. Sex therapy cannot help people with serious relationship problems, depression, or any kind of emotional problem. Here counseling on a regular basis is necessary.

Whether your sex problem is new or long-term, you owe it to yourself to see what can be done about it.

4

SEXUALLY-TRANSMITTED INFECTIONS

Maybe you have never had venereal disease or VD — an infection spread primarily from person to person by sexual intercourse or close physical contact. Even so, you should know the facts: VD is increasing at an alarming rate, especially among sexually active people between 15 and 30. Public health officials are calling it an epidemic or a national health emergency. Moreover, what many people don't realize is that VD is more than just gonorrhea and syphilis. These two infections are the most familiar and the most serious, but there are others. Some of these infections have just begun to be considered venereal or sexually-transmitted infections. The list now includes: gonorrhea, syphilis, non-gonoccocal urethritis (men only), genital herpes, genital warts, crabs, scabies, Trichomonas, Monilia, and Hemophilis vaginitis. And there are about ten other infections, some of which are less common in this country than elsewhere.

The toll of these infections is high. In 1973 about 24,800 cases of infectious syphilis were reported to the Center for Disease Control, a division of the U.S. Public Health Service. By 1977, the number of reported cases had dropped slightly to about 20,400. The gonorrhea statistics are even worse. In 1973 there were about 842,600 cases of gonorrhea. Five years later, in 1977, the number of reported cases had skyrocketed to 1,000,177. Even these dramatic statistics do not tell the entire story, since many cases are not reported. Statisticians estimate that private doctors report anywhere from 10 percent to 25 percent of their cases. By scanning the

Center for Disease Control's most current estimates (Table 2), take a look at how common all these infections are.

You can pretend "It can't happen to me." But the more sexually active you are, the greater your chances of getting one of these infections. Anybody can catch a sexually-transmitted infection. It doesn't matter where you live, if you are rich or poor or in love. Moreover, it doesn't matter who your sexual partner is. These infections can be transmitted from a man to a woman, woman to a man, or between people of the same sex. The best way to protect yourself is to avoid sexual contact with anyone who has a sexually-transmitted infection. But many people who have these infections may not even know it, and one of them could unknowingly give it to you. Though you may have only a few sexual partners, the fact is, your partners may also have other partners.

Protect yourself and stop the spread of sexually-transmitted infections. Know the facts, symptoms, consequences, and what to do.

□ WHEN AND WHERE TO GET HELP

If you think you have been exposed to one of the sexually-transmitted infections — especially gonorrhea or syphilis — don't wait for your yearly exam or for your symptoms to appear or disappear. Often these infections — especially gonorrhea — don't show early symptoms in women. At the first sign of any genital itching, bump, sore, stinging while urinating, heavier than usual discharge, or all these symptoms, get help. Also, remember one attack does not make you immune. You can catch these infections again and again.

Here are some general guidelines:

• Make a checkup appointment right away. If you don't have your own doctor or are uneasy about calling your doctor, you can call any of several places for help. Consult the Yellow Pages under Clinics, Health or Health Department (under your city or state); Planned Parent-

TABLE 2. Estimated Number of Men and Women Affected Yearly by Sexually-Transmitted Infections, 1977

INFECTION	NUMBER OF CASES
Gonorrhea	1,600,000 to 2,000,000
Non-gonococcal Urethritis (men only)	800,000 to 1,000,000
Trichomonas	600,000 to 1,000,000
Genital Warts	200,000 to 400,000
Genital Herpes	150,000 to 200,000
Crabs	100,000 to 200,000
Syphilis	75,000 to 80,000
Scabies	50,000 to 100,000

How sexually-transmitted infections get spread

This may be the "group" you know about

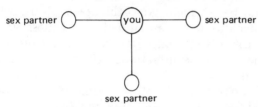

but this is what you're actually in the middle of!

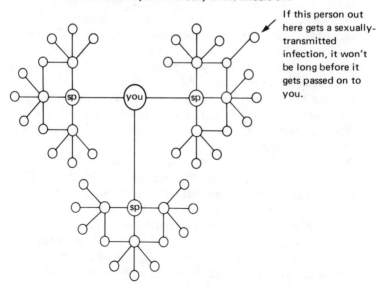

If this person out here gets a sexually-transmitted infection, it won't be long before it gets passed on to you.

(Adapted from the American Social Health Association, 1977.)

51

hood; local VD Clinic (in community health centers and hospitals); Board of Health; and State Department of Public Health (Division of Communicable and Venereal Diseases). If you have trouble locating a place, you can call the national VD hotline, Operation Venus. (See Readings and Resources.) They can help you find a place for diagnosis and treatment nearest home.

- Diagnosis and treatment will be strictly confidential. Your school, college, or employer will not be notified. In almost every state, minors don't need the consent of their parents for diagnosis and treatment. If you are in doubt about your state laws, call your local health department or Operation Venus for the current regulations in your state.

- If you think you have caught gonorrhea or syphilis, ask for a special checkup for these infections. Unless you specifically ask for this checkup, you will not automatically receive one for these infections. Meanwhile, don't have sex until you know.

- Home remedies *do not* work. Most people who try to treat themselves eventually end up seeking medical help. Don't try to treat yourself by using a friend's medication or an antibiotic left over from an old prescription. Get proper medical treatment. Sometimes symptoms disappear before you are completely cured. So you need to keep using your medication for the prescribed time to prevent another flare-up.

- During treatment, don't have sex with anyone until you have proof of cure. This varies from infection to infection, so ask the doctor when to schedule follow-up visits after treatment.

- One of the best ways to stop the spread of these infections is to have your sexual partners go for tests. If you develop a sexually-transmitted infection, notify *all* your recent sexual contacts, either personally or through a casefinder. Your place of treatment will probably ask you for names and phone numbers of your sexual partners. Casefinders make every effort to handle such matters without embarrassment for everyone. (This is done without revealing your name.)

☐ GONORRHEA

Whether called the clap, a dose, a strain, the runs, the morning whites, or drip, gonorrhea ranks as the second most common communicable disease in the United States. The common cold is first. Once thought to be a disease of big cities, gonorrhea has moved to the suburbs, small towns, rural areas, colleges, and high schools. It is prevalent everywhere. Not only is it currently out of control in the United States, but public health officials estimate that, worldwide, there are 100 million cases of gonorrhea each year. Moreover, the number is rising. Experts further estimate that there are close to one million American women who don't know they have gonorrhea. Why? Because gonorrhea doesn't cause symptoms in nearly three out of five women.

Caused by the bacteria *Neisseria gonorrhoeae*, gonorrhea is almost always transmitted by sexual intercourse. This is because the gonococcus organism requires a moist mucus-like surface for survival, like the throat, vagina, cervix, urethra, or rectum. Depending on how you have sex, it can be passed to or from the penis, vagina, mouth, or anus. Rarely can you get gonorrhea from such things as toilet seats. However, newborn infants can acquire a potentially blinding infection of the eyes (gonococcal conjunctivitis) while passing through the mother's infected birth canal. To prevent this and other eye infections, doctors place silver nitrate or penicillin drops in the eyes of all infants immediately after birth. This precaution is almost 100 percent effective.

If you think you have caught gonorrhea—or a sexual partner notifies you—don't wait for your yearly exam or for symptoms to show up. Make an appointment right away. If diagnosed early, gonorrhea can be treated easily. Untreated, it can cause serious complications in both sexes.

Common Symptoms

Nearly 60 percent to 70 percent of all *women* never notice any early warning signs or symptoms until weeks or months after exposure. Frequently, the first sign of a woman's infection is gonorrhea in one of her male sex partners. These asymptomatic women remain "carriers." They unknowingly spread gonorrhea to their sexual contacts while their own infection progresses. The remaining women often develop mild, easily-overlooked symptoms. About a week to ten days after sexual contact the infection, which usually begins in the cervix, causes an irritating, creamy, rather thick vaginal discharge. Inflammation of the urethra (urinary channel) may cause pain or burning while urinating. (Many women mistake this symptom for a bladder infection.) A few women also have a trichomonal infection that causes a foamy, white or greenish-yellow vaginal discharge and severe genital itching, burning, and soreness.

Among *men*, about 90 percent develop obvious signs about two to five days after sexual contact. At first, there is a thin, clear, discharge that rapidly becomes heavy, creamy, and thick. The next sign may be only a drop of pus at the end of the penis when arising. This accounts for the nickname, "morning whites." Most men also feel pain and burning while urinating, sometimes described as "pissing pins and needles." Other signs to watch out for in uncircumcised men are irritation and redness under the foreskin of the penis. The remaining men who don't develop symptoms remain "carriers." Like women, they never notice any early warning signs of gonorrhea until weeks or months after exposure. Unfortunately, recent studies show that the number of asymptomatic men is increasing.

For both *men and women*, early gonorrhea does not always confine itself to the reproductive system and urinary tract. As a result of oral sex, infections of the mouth and throat are common. While it is possible to have an oral infection without symptoms, some people develop a sore throat and low-grade fever several days after sex. Additionally, infection of the anus can result from anal sex, careless wiping with toilet tissue, or from feminine napkins. On occasion anal sex causes symptoms, so be alert for any discharge from the anus, painful or bloody bowel movements, or pain in the rectum or anus.

If ignored or unnoticed, these common symptoms of gonorrhea can disappear without treatment. Disappearance of symptoms means only that the gonococcus organisms have moved to another part of the body. It does not mean that your gonorrhea has gone away or cured itself.

Less Common Symptoms and Complications

Untreated or improperly treated gonorrhea can cause serious complications.

In *women*, the gonococcus bacteria can spread beyond the cervix to the reproductive system and cause a painful, serious infection known as pelvic inflammatory disease. (IUD users are at much higher risk for developing this infection than other women with gonorrhea.) This usually happens during or immediately after the first menstrual period, when the infection can spread quickly up the uterus. The first — and sometimes only — sign of gonorrhea passing into the uterus is a change in the menstrual periods. Periods may begin too soon, last longer than usual, or be especially heavy. Moreover, cramping may be more severe. The real trouble begins when the gonococcus organisms spread from the uterus to the Fallopian tubes, causing inflammation and the development of pus within the tubal passageways (salpingitis). From the Fallopian tubes, the infection can then spread to the ovaries and into the pelvic cavity (peritonitis). If early symptoms were minimal, ignored, or even absent, pelvic inflammatory disease usually produces real distress. Lower abdominal pain during or after the menstrual period, an obvious discharge, fever, chills, and occasionally vomiting are among the common symptoms. These symptoms demand prompt medical attention. A delay of a day or two may well make the difference between complete recovery and permanent tubal damage.

Reports show that about 15 percent to 25 percent of all women become sterile as a result of tubal scarring and blockage from only one attack of pelvic inflammatory disease. Another disturbing aspect of pelvic inflammatory disease is its tendency to flare-up or recur. With each additional attack, the risk of becoming sterile increases. In addition, if an egg from one of the ovaries enters a scarred tube and becomes fertilized, pregnancy can develop in the tube instead of the uterus. Such pregnancies (ectopic) are dangerous since the tubes are too small to support a pregnancy. (If you miss one period and develop other signs of pregnancy, go to a doctor for a pregnancy test.) Lastly, women with active pelvic inflammatory disease who develop a pregnancy in the uterus experience high rates of miscarriage, premature births, and stillbirths.

In *men*, untreated gonorrhea can spread up the urethra to the reproductive system. If the sperm ducts become infected, sterility can result. Since obvious symptoms usually appear early in men, complications from gonorrhea are rare.

Even though gonorrhea is usually limited to the reproductive system, it can affect other parts of the body. Once gonococcus organisms spread into the blood stream, gonorrhea can be responsible for arthritis, heart lesions, and even meningitis, to name just a few problems seen in both men and women. While these complications are quite rare, they are slightly more common in women than in men.

Diagnosis

If you think you have caught gonorrhea, go to your doctor or clinic promptly and ask for a special checkup for gonorrhea. Unless you specifically ask for this checkup, you will not automatically receive it.

Currently there are two diagnostic tests for gonorrhea: the smear (Gram stain) and culture. The simplest is the smear test. A small amount of discharge from the cervix, penis, throat, or anus is spread onto a slide, stained with special dyes, and examined under a microscope. The smear test is not always accurate. Approximately five percent of men and 40 percent of women with gonorrhea have "false-negative" results. For this reason, most doctors rely on the culture test for women. This test is highly accurate if discharge is taken from each of three places: the cervix, urethra, and anus. After growing and observing the discharge in a special laboratory medium for 48 hours, the gonococcus organisms can easily be detected.

To be sure of accurate results, don't douche or take any medications before your test.

Treatment

Treatment usually consists of two injections of penicillin. In addition, many doctors routinely give an oral medication (probenecid) to increase the penicillin's effectiveness. Ampicillin, an oral medication related to penicillin, may also be used. Men or women allergic to these drugs may be given either of two antibiotics, tetracycline or spectinomycin. However, treatment varies. Over ten years ago, 1,200,000 units of penicillin would cure gonorrhea. Now, it takes four times that amount and sometimes more. Though the *right* amount of antibiotic still works, certain new strains of gonorrhea are slowly developing resistance to penicillin and other antibiotics. Even so, these new strains of "penicillin resistant gonorrhea" are still curable with the right type and amount of antibiotic.

Treatment of pelvic inflammatory disease — a complication of gonorrhea — varies with the degree of infection. Mild forms usually require only antibiotics and bedrest. Certain severe or recurrent cases may, however, require hysterectomy. This is because pelvic inflammatory disease may actually be life-threatening. (See Chapter 5.)

Even though symptoms begin to clear quickly after treatment, you need to keep using your medication for the prescribed time. Don't try to treat yourself by using a friend's medication or an antibiotic left over from an old prescription.

Proof of cure depends on two to three negative cultures at one-week intervals after treatment. Of course, positive cultures require further treatment. As for prevention, avoiding contact with infected sexual partners is the only sure way. Right now there is no vaccine. One attack of gonorrhea does not make you immune. You can get gonorrhea again and again.

☐ SYPHILIS

Casually referred to as siff, Old Joe, the lues, the sore, or bad blood, syphilis is a serious, terrible disease. In fact, it ranks as the most potentially devastating of the sexually-transmitted infections. Unlike gonorrhea, it is not nearly as widespread. Syphilis is not as common as gonorrhea, but this fact does not undermine its seriousness. Left untreated during the early stages, syphilis can go into hiding and not show any outward signs. Slowly and insidiously syphilis can reappear years later, with destructive consequences.

Caused by a corkscrew-shaped bacteria or spirochete called *Treponema pallidum*, syphilis is almost always transmitted by sexual intercourse. This is because spirochetes require a warm, moist surface like the vulva, penis, throat, vagina, or anus for survival. Depending on how you have sex, it can be passed to or from the penis, vagina, mouth, or anus. Spirochetes can also twist and burrow their way through cuts or breaks in the skin on the finger, hand, leg, breast, or around the mouth, for example. Moreover, even though syphilis is not hereditary, pregnant women can transmit syphilis to their unborn infants.

If you think you have caught syphilis, or your partner notifies you, don't wait for your yearly exam or for symptoms to show up. Make an appointment with your doctor or clinic right away. If diagnosed early, syphilis can be treated easily. Untreated, it can cause serious complications in both men and women.

Common Symptoms

Anywhere from ten to ninety days following exposure — with three weeks as the average — symptoms of *primary syphilis* can appear. The first sign is usually a chancre (pronounced "shanker"). It may look like a pimple, blister, or bump that becomes an open sore full or highly infectious spirochetes. The chancre is so infectious that this is the most contagious stage of syphilis. Ranging in size from very tiny to the size of a dime, chancres develop at the site of infection, where the spirochetes enter the body. In the *man*, it usually appears on the tip of the penis but can occur inside the urethra (urinary channel) or under the foreskin of uncircumcised men. In the *woman*, it most often appears on the vulva or opening of the vagina. Occasionally, it may be high up on the cervix or vagina and not be noticeable at all. In both *men and women*, chancres can appear on or in the mouth, anus, leg, arm, or anywhere the spirochete takes hold.

If the chancre is unnoticed or ignored, it will go away. With or without treatment, this sign of primary syphilis always goes away within two to six weeks. For this reason, many people with syphilis are fooled. They think their problem has gone away. Nothing could be further from the truth. The spirochetes are still inside the body, traveling through the blood stream.

Less Common Symptoms and Complications

If primary syphilis is not diagnosed and treated, it *may* progress through three other stages.

In about six weeks, but as long as six months after the chancre goes away, the next set of symptoms — called *secondary syphilis* — comes along. During this stage a skin rash, made up of many small, red hard bumps, may cover the body or appear only on the palms of the hands or the soles of the feet. The rash may be coupled with flu-like symptoms (tiredness, fever, sore throat, headache, and a general aching in the muscles and joints) in addition to hair falling out in patches. Even without treatment, these symptoms disappear after a few weeks. Meanwhile, the spirochetes are now in the blood stream traveling to other parts of the body.

Only during the primary and secondary stages, which can last up to two years, can you transmit syphilis to other people. An exception is the pregnant woman with untreated syphilis who may transmit syphilis to her unborn baby indefinitely. (This is why the law requires every prospective mother to receive a blood test for syphilis.) After the third month of pregnancy, a pregnant woman with syphilis can pass the disease on to her fetus. Every month that passes without treatment increases the chance of complications for the unborn infant. Once the fetus becomes infected, syphilis can cause miscarriage, stillbirth, or a live infant with congenital syphilis. Fortunately, diagnosis and treatment before the third month of pregnancy will prevent the fetus from developing syphilis and its complications. Treatment after this time and before birth will cure the child. It cannot, however, reverse damage already done. Congenital syphilis may involve deformities in the bones, skin, teeth, eyes, and other parts of the nervous system.

Untreated secondary syphilis is followed by *latent syphilis.* This stage, which may last a few years or a lifetime, is without outward signs. There is no way to determine the length of the latent stage. But, in one out of three people with untreated latent syphilis, the spirochetes continue to spread and multiply in certain parts of the body. During this time the spirochetes may begin their damage in the heart, brain, and spinal cord. When this happens, the disease is no longer latent and the signs of *late syphilis* appear. Complications of late syphilis may involve mental illness, blindness, heart disease, or even death. With current methods of diagnosis and treatment, very few men or women ever reach the late stage of syphilis.

Diagnosis

If you think you have caught syphilis, go to your doctor or clinic promptly, and ask for a special checkup for syphilis. Unless you specifically ask for this checkup, you will not automatically receive it.

Syphilis has been called the "Great Imitator" because so many of its symptoms mimic other diseases such as psoriasis, drug rashes, mononucleosis, and even cancer. For this reason, the doctor cannot depend on your symptoms alone. Medical diagnosis of syphilis depends on your symptoms, history of exposure, and positive laboratory tests.

Currently, there are two types of laboratory tests for syphilis: the darkfield exam and blood tests. If a chancre is present, your doctor takes some fluid from the sore and checks for the presence of spirochetes under a special "dark-field" microscope. Anyone suspected of having syphilis is also given a blood test whether or not the darkfield test is positive. Also, most states legally require blood tests for couples who apply for a marriage license; pregnant women; people donating blood; and anyone who is admitted to a hospital or enters the Armed Forces.

Blood tests serve to confirm the diagnosis of syphilis, especially when symptoms are confusing or absent. Rather than detecting the presence of spirochetes, they work by detecting antibodies that the body produces to fight off the spirochetes. The most common blood test is the VDRL (Venereal Disease Research Laboratory) test. It is fairly reliable (four to six weeks after exposure), easy to perform, and inexpensive. If there are any doubts about the results of the VDRL, a second test, the FTA-ABS (fluorescent treponemal antibody absorption) test can be performed. This test is more accurate in cases of early syphilis.

To be sure of accurate results, don't take any medications or put any cream or ointment on your sore (if present) before your exam.

Treatment

Treatment of primary and secondary syphilis usually consists of two injections of penicillin. Latent and late syphilis require larger doses of antibiotics. Men or women allergic to penicillin may be given either of three antibiotics, tetracycline, erythromycin, or cephaloridine. While proper treatment will cure all stages of syphilis, it cannot reverse damage already done.

Even though symptoms begin to clear quickly after treatment, you need to keep using your medication for the prescribed time. Don't try to treat yourself by using a friend's medication or an antibiotic left over from an old prescription.

Proof of cure depends on several follow-up exams and blood tests after treatment. If you were treated for primary or secondary syphilis, you should see a doctor one month after treatment and then once every three months for at least a year. If treatment was adequate, a positive VDRL blood test usually becomes negative within six to twelve months for primary syphilis and twelve to eighteen months for secondary syphilis. More frequent follow-up exams are necessary for latent and late syphilis.

As for prevention, avoiding contact with infected sexual partners is the only sure way. Right now there is no vaccine. One attack of syphilis does not make you immune. You can get syphilis again and again.

☐ GENITAL HERPES

Herpes (pronounced "Hur-peez") is the common term for two viral infections currently existing in epidemic levels in the United States. One form — herpes simplex virus type 1 — is best known as the cause of fever blisters and cold sores on or around the lips. Another form — herpes simplex virus type 2 — almost always occurs below the waist, especially in and around the genital area. Most genital herpes infections are caused by contact with the type 2 virus during sexual intercourse. However, in an estimated five percent of all cases, doctors find type 1 and type 2 in reverse areas, probably as a result of oral sex.

Symptoms

About a week after exposure to the herpes virus, the first symptoms may be burning, itching, or tingling in the genital area. These symptoms then develop into one or several groups of small, red, painful bumps or blisters. In *women*, the blisters usually occur on the external genital area, but may affect the thighs, anus, or the buttocks. Painless blisters may also occur on the cervix and vagina. In *men*, blisters usually appear on the penis. Several days later, the blisters go away or rupture to form painful sores. During this stage, you can easily spread the infection to other areas of your body as well as to your sexual partners. Moreover, these open sores can become infected by bacteria. Within a week or so, these sores eventually scab and heal.

The first attack of herpes type 2 may last up to a month. In addition to the blisters, some people have fever, headaches, swelling of the lymph nodes inside the thighs, and overall weakness. After the first attack, the virus does not leave the body. Even after symptoms disappear, the virus does not. Instead, it goes into hiding and continues to live in the body in a noncontagious stage.

Perhaps the most disturbing aspect of herpes is its tendency to flare-up or recur in about 70 percent of all men and women. This means that there is no limit to the number of times you can get it. You may not have any symptoms for months or years and then herpes may appear at any time. Such occurrences as fever, sunburn, and physical or emotional stress can trigger recurrences. Also, some women experience occasional battles with herpes about a week before their menstrual period. Fortunately, recurrent attacks are usually milder and shorter. As time goes by, herpes seems to recur less often after the first attack.

Complications

During pregnancy, women with an active herpes type 2 infection may miscarry or deliver early. Also, if the newborn gets herpes while passing through the birth canal, the baby may recover completely or develop a potentially fatal brain infection. The risk to the baby is greatest when the mother is having her *first* attack of herpes — rather than a *recurrent* one — within four weeks of delivery. Fortunately, women with a history of herpes rarely transmit the infection to their baby, unless open sores are present at delivery. When herpes is present at delivery, obstetricians can reduce the risk of complications by delivering the baby by cesarean section to avoid its exposure to the virus.

Secondly, medical scientists suspect a possible relationship between herpes type 2 and cervical cancer. While no cause and effect relationship has been established, researchers report that women with herpes type 2 of the cervix are eight times more likely to develop cervical cancer than women without herpes. If you have herpes type 2, have regular exams with a Pap test every six months. Cervical conditions diagnosed in their early stages are usually 100 percent curable.

Diagnosis

Medical diagnosis of herpes is often difficult. This is because many men and women don't see a doctor until late in the infection when scabs have already formed over the blisters. It turns out that the dry crusted scabs, which develop in the final stage, are the mirror image of the chancre of syphilis and are often mistaken for it.

To insure an accurate diagnosis, see a doctor when your symptoms are in the blister stage. Diagnosis is often determined by inspection of the blisters. It can also be made by microscopic examination of fluid from the blisters. Apart from this, diagnosis is best made by growing the virus in a special laboratory culture or testing for the presence of antibodies with a special blood test. These last two laboratory tests, however, are only available in well-equipped hospitals.

Treatment

At present there is no cure for herpes. Antibiotics, which successfully cure most of the other sexually-transmitted infections, are of little help in fighting off the herpes virus. Instead, treatment is aimed at the relief of symptoms. Sitzbaths or wet dressings of cool water two to three times a day can offer relief until the infection runs its course. In general, you should avoid creams and ointments. If the sores are especially painful, a pain-relieving cream (such as Xylocaine) may be helpful. Warm baths, gently washing the sores with a germ-killing soap (such as Betadine), good genital hygiene, and wearing loose-fitting cotton underpants can help prevent bacterial infection. (If infection occurs, sulfa creams are available with a prescription.) Be sure to avoid sexual intercourse during a herpes outbreak. This will help prevent irritation and transmitting the infection to your sexual partners.

More recently, several methods of treatment have been tried but with little evidence that they are of value. For example, repeated smallpox vaccines have been tried to prevent recurrences. The "dye-and-light" method has been tried by many doctors. This involves applying a special dye to the herpes sores and then exposing this painted area to light for about 15 minutes. It remains a highly controversial type of treatment in that there are questions about the safety and value of this method. Moreover, several case-control studies have shown that this method provides few, if any, benefits. Right now researchers are working on more promising ways to treat herpes.

☐ GENITAL WARTS

Genital warts or *Condyloma acuminata* are here in epidemic proportions. Until recently these virus-induced growths were called venereal or gonorrheal warts because most doctors thought they were transmitted only by sexual intercourse. Though warts are usually transmitted by sexual intercourse, pregnancy, the birth control pill, excessive vaginal discharge, and poor genital hygiene can also encourage their growth.

Symptoms

One to three months after exposure, tiny pinkish-tan growths can appear anywhere on the genitals. In *women*, they usually appear near the vaginal opening, but can also occur on the vaginal lips, vagina, cervix, and around the anus. In *men*, warts usually occur on the tip of the penis, and less often under the foreskin or on the shaft of the penis.

At first there may be one or several warts, discharge, and

itching. However, if kept moist by excessive discharge, warts can flourish and grow. Especially during pregnancy, warts can mushroom into cauliflower-like masses.

Diagnosis

Medical diagnosis is simple. A doctor can diagnose genital warts by inspecting them. Laboratory tests are rarely necessary.

Treatment

Though startling in appearance, treatment is easy. Small warts can be dried up with an anti-wart solution (podophyllin). Warts may require several treatments at your doctor's office or clinic. Six hours after treatment make sure to wash off the medication, since it may cause chemical burns. If the warts are large, hot cauterization or even minor surgery may be necessary.

If you are plagued with repeated episodes of genital warts, wearing cotton underpants and avoiding clothing that traps moisture (nylon underwear and pantyhose, for example) may help. If you use the birth control pill, you may have to stop temporarily until the warts clear up. And, if warts appear during pregnancy, a complete cure may have to wait until after delivery.

☐ CRABS

Pubic lice or *Pediculosis pubis* exist almost in epidemic proportions. Usually transmitted by sexual intercourse or very close physical contact, you can sometimes catch them from infected articles such as clothing, sheets, blankets, sleeping bags, or toilet seats. Once this parasite latches on, it buries its head inside a pubic hair follicle and proceeds to cause almost intolerable itching. Scratching does not bring relief, but can occasionally carry the crabs to other hairy parts of the body such as the thighs, underarms, and face.

Symptoms

If you develop a maddening pubic itch and can spot any other telltale signs such as tiny white or rust-colored specks in your pubic hair, don't panic. As loathsome as pubic crabs may be, they don't carry any horrible disease.

Diagnosis

Medical diagnosis is made by locating the crabs or their eggs on the pubic hairs. Each crab, though tiny, is visible without a microscope.

Treatment

First of all, don't shave your pubic hair or try to treat yourself with something as ineffective as soap and water. Two medications which work rapidly and effectively are gamma benzene hexachloride (Kwell), a prescription lotion; or A-200 Pyrinate, a lotion available in drugstores without a prescription.

After treatment, you should change your clothes and bedclothes. Crabs die within 24 hours after separation from the body, but their eggs can live for about two weeks. This means that previously used bedclothes, towels, and other articles are safe after two weeks without use. You can use anything laundered in boiling water or dry-cleaned immediately. Moreover, remember to scrub the toilet seat.

☐ SCABIES

Commonly called the seven-year itch, scabies — caused by a small parasitic mite — are transmitted the same way as crabs.

Symptoms

Scabies cause severe itching and red bumps or lines wherever the mite burrows under the skin. This usually happens between the fingers, on the wrists, underarms, chest, thighs, male genitals, and occasionally on a woman's genitals. Itching, especially at night, usually begins about four to six weeks after contact with an infected person. Scratching does not bring relief but may cause infection and further complicate the problem.

Diagnosis

Medical diagnosis is made after physical examination or by obtaining a mite from inside a burrow and identifying it under a microscope.

Treatment

Treatment is the same as that for crabs. After treatment, you should change your clothes and bedclothes. Be sure to wash or dry-clean previously used clothes and bedclothes. Moreover, remember to scrub the toilet seat.

☐ TRICHOMONAS

Better known as "trich" or TV for short, a one-celled parasite causes this infection. Trichomonas can live harmlessly in a woman's body without causing infection or discharge. And then something, such as a menstrual period or lowered resistance, can trigger a trichomonal infection. Trichomonas can also survive for several hours on moist objects such as toilet seats, wash clothes, towels, and wet bathing suits. Yet sexual contact is probably the major means of transmission.

Moreover, some men unknowingly harbor the Trichomonas organism in their urinary tract or under their foreskin (if uncircumcised). Men, however, usually don't have symptoms. They often transfer Trichomonas from one woman to another without ever developing symptoms themselves. This is one of the reasons why Trichomonas is so widespread.

Symptoms

Symptoms usually appear four to twenty days after contact with the organism. Frequently, the infection produces a foamy, white, or greenish-yellow vaginal discharge that smells unpleasant. It usually causes vaginal soreness, itching, burning, and, less frequently, a rash along the inner thighs. Sexual intercourse during this time is often painful. Left untreated, Trichomonas can spread to the urinary tract and cause an even more serious infection. Though most men don't have symptoms, those that do may notice a slight discharge and itching on their penis.

Diagnosis

Medical diagnosis is confirmed by microscopically examining the discharge or growing the parasite in a special laboratory culture. (If you have a Pap test taken when you have Trichomonas, the organism can make the cells appear abnormal, often resulting in a "false-positive" Pap result.)

Treatment

Until 1960 there was no adequate treatment for Trichomonas, though various douches and local medications were tried with little success. This is because Trichomonas may hide in places such as the bladder, where local treatment can't get to the organisms. Currently the most effective treatment is an oral prescription drug metronidazale (Flagyl). If your partner also receives Flagyl and you avoid sexual intercourse (or have your partner use a condom) during treatment, the chances of cure approach 100 percent. Itching and discharge usually disappear in several days. Even so, you need to keep using the medication for the prescribed time to avoid another flare-up. Flagyl side effects may include: nausea, diarrhea, or a bad taste in the mouth. If you have any of the following conditions, you should not use Flagyl, but another medication: pregnancy; breast-feeding; certain diseases of the blood and central nervous system. Also, avoid alcohol while taking Flagyl. Even a glass of beer can cause nausea, cramps, and dizziness.

Since 1960 millions of women have used Flagyl without any dangerous side effects. Since the early 1970s, several research studies have reported that laboratory mice and rats fed high doses of Flagyl all their lives developed a significantly higher number of cancers (especially of the lungs) than animals that did not receive Flagyl. In 1974 a Ralph Nader consumer protection group called for the removal of Flagyl from the market because of the cancer risk. Since then, there has been much publicity about Flagyl and the so-called "cancer risk." Review of all available medical information shows that there is no evidence whatever that Flagyl can cause cancer in humans even though it causes cancer in laboratory animals. This all means that Flagyl, if properly used, continues to be a safe, highly-effective treatment for Trichomonas.

☐ MONILIA

Also known as vaginal thrush or Candida, a yeast-like fungus causes Monilia. A normal inhabitant of many healthy vaginas, women and men also harbor Monilia in their mouths, intestines, between their buttocks, and other parts of the body. This organism also lives harmlessly in urine, semen, and under the foreskins of uncircumcised men. Unless certain conditions such as pregnancy, the birth control pill, diabetes, antibiotics, or excessive genital moisture, favor its growth, Monilia remains harmless.

Monilia can be transmitted in several ways. For example,

it can travel from the anus along the surface of a menstrual pad or from careless wiping with toilet tissue. Monilia can also be transmitted by vaginal, anal, or oral-genital sex. Oral thrush — inflammation and soreness of the mouth, tongue, or pharynx — from oral sex is rare. Also, a Monilia infection during pregnancy and delivery can affect the newborn with a similar infection of the mouth called thrush. Thrush in the newborn can be easily treated and will leave no aftereffects.

Symptoms

Monilia usually brings on intense itching and swelling of the vagina and vulva, and, less frequently, a rash along the inner thighs. If you have this infection, you may also notice a white or cream-colored discharge that looks something like cottage cheese and smells a little like baking bread. Sexual intercourse may be painful and urination frequent. Many men don't have symptoms, while others may notice itching, irritation, or a slight discharge of the penis after intercourse.

Diagnosis

Medical diagnosis is confirmed by microscopically examining the discharge or growing the fungus in a special laboratory culture.

Treatment

There is no adequate way to treat Monilia yourself. Though sitting in a bathtub with cool water and applying wet compresses can help relieve the itching, you must see a doctor for treatment. Treatment usually consists of inserting antibiotic cream or suppositories into the vagina for about two weeks. Though itching usually disappears in several days, you need to keep using the medication for the prescribed time. If your symptoms are severe or if they persist, other types of treatment include oral antibiotics or having your vagina, cervix, and vulva painted with gentian violet solution.

☐ HEMOPHILUS VAGINITIS

Until the mid-1950s, doctors called all other vaginal infections "nonspecific vaginitis." But it is now known that most of these infections are caused by a specific bacteria: Hemophilus vaginalis. The remainder, caused by other bacteria, are called nonspecific vaginitis.

Like Trichomonas, Hemophilus is often transmitted by sexual intercourse. Yet forgotten tampons, anal-vaginal sex, vaginal spermicides, feminine deodorant sprays, and too-frequent douching can also cause this infection.

Symptoms

Symptoms usually appear five to ten days after sexual contact with an infected person. They are similar to those of Trichomonas, though the discharge tends to be grayish-white and especially foul-smelling.

Diagnosis

Medical diagnosis is confirmed by microscopically examining the discharge.

Treatment

Doctors tend to start off treating this infection with vaginal creams or suppositories. Yet new studies suggest that metronidazole (Flagyl) works best for this condition. If your infection persists—as it sometimes can—contact your doctor about treatment for both you and partner. This infection can be difficult to cure, if not treated properly.

☐ PREVENTION

If you are sexually active, there is no foolproof way to avoid getting a sexually-transmitted infection. There are only two guaranteed preventives. Avoiding sex is one sure way. Similarly, when two people both free of a sexually-transmitted infection have sex only with each other, they can be sure of not getting one of these infections. The ultimate preventive is, of course, vaccines. Right now there is no immunization against sexually-transmitted infections. But researchers are testing trial vaccines.

Though you can't reduce your odds of getting a sexually-transmitted infection to zero, here are some ways to minimize your risk:

- If you are sexually active, have regular checkups for sexually-transmitted infections, especially gonorrhea and syphilis. (Ask your doctor or clinic for a special checkup several times a year.)
- Have your male partner use a condom. To be effective, it must be worn during the entire time his penis is in contact with your genitals, anus, or mouth. If used correctly, the condom provides complete protection against gonorrhea, Trichomonas, Monilia, and Hemophilus vaginitis and good protection against syphilis, herpes, and genital warts.
- Washing hands and genitals with soap and water before and after sex might help remove some organisms.
- Urinating immediately after sex might flush out some organisms.
- Interestingly, many contraceptive foams, jellies, and creams — if inserted before intercourse — provide some protection against gonorrhea and syphilis.

- You may have heard that the birth control pill and IUD can prevent sexually-transmitted infections. It's not true. They can prevent nothing but pregnancy. In fact, the Pill (through certain chemical changes in the vagina) and especially the IUD (through menstrual changes) can actually increase the chances of getting gonorrhea.
- Examine your partner's penis before it becomes erect. If your partner has a cloudy discharge or any unusual sores, don't have sex. (Since men and women can unknowingly have a sexually-transmitted infection, the only sure protection is a condom.)

   Here are some additional ways to help prevent Trichomonas, Monilia, and Hemophilus vaginitis: sexually-transmitted infections that may have causes other than sexual contact.

- Wash your genitals and buttocks regularly. When you wash, be sure to clean inside the folds of your vulva as well as around your rectum where bacteria hide and grow. Also be sure to rinse the soap, since it can cause itching and irritation. After washing, pat your genitals dry and keep them fairly dry. Use only your own towel and wash cloth, and avoid harsh soaps.
- Wear clean, cotton underpants. Tight girdles, pantyhose, nylon underpants, and even pants that have a snug crotch tend to trap moisture—an environment for bacteria to grow.
- Wipe your anus from front to back to avoid carrying bacteria to your vagina.
- In public bathrooms, flush the toilet before you sit down to help rid any organisms that may be lurking in the water. Also, use disposable toilet seat covers or put toilet paper on the seat. Remember to wash your hands afterward.
- If you are plagued with repeated Monilia infections, sometimes cutting back on carbohydrates, sugar, and alcohol helps. Also, get tested for diabetes.

5

OTHER HEALTH PROBLEMS

☐ **BLADDER INFECTION**

At one time or another, many women develop an attack of cystitis, inflammation and infection of the bladder. This problem is usually caused by bacteria that enter the bladder through the urethra, and women — rather than men — are more prone to cystitis. For every ten women that get cystitis, one man develops it. Since the woman's urethra (channel that takes urine from the bladder to outside the body) is only an inch and a half long, the bacteria have a short distance to travel to infect the bladder. (The man's urethra is about eight inches long.) And, if you add other factors, the chances of getting cystitis increase. For example, during pregnancy and right after childbirth and surgery such as hysterectomy, the risk of developing cystitis is higher than usual. Sometimes cystitis is related to sexual intercourse. For example, it can occur after prolonged sexual intercourse or in women who have just begun having sexual relations. This explains the nickname "honeymoon" cystitis.

If you suddenly have to urinate a lot, and this burns and stings — though hardly anything comes out — you probably have cystitis. Cystitis may also cause a sense of pressure or heaviness just above the pubic bone. Severe infections can cause blood in the urine. And yet symptoms can be misleading. You can't blame all painful urination on bladder infections. Many of the sexually-transmitted infections in Chapter 4 can easily mimic cystitis. So get prompt medical diagnosis and treatment.

Your doctor or clinic will ask you for a urine sample; therefore drink several glasses of water before the exam. Diagnosis involves microscopic examination of your urine for the presence of bacteria. Laboratory results take about a day or two. In any event, most doctors start treatment right away with sulfisoxazole (Gantrisin, for example). But there are many other types of medications.

If you develop cystitis, here are some helpful pointers:

- Whether or not your symptoms disappear within several days, you need to keep taking your medication for the prescribed time. Anything short of this only invites another flare-up.
- Drink plenty of water — about ten glasses a day — during treatment. This helps keep your urine diluted and the bacteria flushed out of your bladder.
- Avoid drinking coffee, tea, and alcohol during treatment since these liquids can irritate the bladder.
- Urinate when you feel like it. Avoiding urination is bad for the bladder.
- Urinate before and after sexual intercourse. In addition, drink several glasses of water after intercourse, especially if you tend to get recurrent bouts of cystitis. Also, use K-Y jelly or vaginal spermicide to keep your vagina lubricated. If intercourse is painful, avoid it until you are cured.
- Return for a follow-up exam three to four weeks after treatment, or earlier if your symptoms persist after treatment.
- If you are plagued with recurrent bouts of cystitis, further diagnostic tests may be necessary. Drink ten or more glasses of water a day and see a doctor as soon as your symptoms develop. Untreated bladder infections can cause serious kidney complications.

☐ CERVICITIS

Cervicitis — inflammation and/or infection of the cervix — is one of the most common problems in gynecology. In fact, it is so common that almost all women who deliver a baby develop some degree of cervicitis. This is because stretching of the cervix during labor and delivery causes inflammation and rawness at the opening of the cervix. When this happens, the cervix can become infected. Almost anything else that exposes the cervix to irritation can also cause cervicitis, including: sexually-transmitted infections; poor personal hygiene (such as anal-vaginal sex); too-frequent douching with irritating solutions; forgotten tampons and diaphragms.

In many women — especially those who have just delivered a baby — cervicitis is so mild it doesn't cause symptoms or require treatment. Other women may notice an irritating, unpleasant smelling, white or yellow vaginal discharge. Less common symptoms may include: low back pain; pain during intercourse and menstruation; and spotting between menstrual periods (especially after intercourse or douching).

Diagnosis and treatment are simple. Diagnosis involves a Pap test and possibly removal of a small amount of tissue from the cervix for microscopic examination (biopsy). How cervicitis is treated depends on its severity. Mild cases usually don't require treatment. When treatment is necessary, it usually consists of antibiotics. Sometimes cryosurgery or hot cauterization is called for. In cryosurgery, infected areas on the cervix are frozen and destroyed. In hot cauterization, infected areas on the cervix are burned and destroyed.

Cervicitis itself is a fairly harmless condition. Left untreated, it can increase the chances of developing infertility.

☐ ENDOMETRIOSIS

The special tissue that lines the uterus (endometrium) normally confines itself to inside the uterus. In some women, however, the endometrial tissue grows outside the uterus, often on the surfaces of the uterus, ovaries, and Fallopian tubes. It attaches itself less often to other pelvic organs. When this happens it is called endometriosis. While it is difficult to make estimates about how many women develop this condition, studies show that about one out of five women undergoing surgery for gynecologic conditions have endometriosis.

Though some women harbor the notion that endometriosis is a form of cancer, it's not true. This noncancerous condition can, however, cause major problems. Usually affecting women between the ages of 25 and 45 — especially women who have never delivered a baby — it can be a major cause of painful menstrual periods, infertility, and severe pain during sexual intercourse. Fortunately, after menopause endometriosis goes away by itself.

The cause of this bizarre condition is not fully understood. Even so, it is most likely the result of tiny shreds of endometrial tissue finding their way through the Fallopian tubes into the pelvic cavity during menstrual periods. Each month these misplaced bits of tissue behave much like the lining of the uterus. Under the influence of ovarian hormones, the areas of endometriosis actually swell, thicken, and bleed every month just like the lining of the uterus.

Symptoms of endometriosis usually begin in the late twenties or early thirties. After years of relatively pain-free menstrual periods, most women with endometriosis notice increasingly painful menstrual periods. Many women develop a nagging soreness in the abdomen and lower back. The location of the endometriosis can sometimes cause other women to have pain during sexual intercourse, especially during the week before the menstrual period. Moreover, many women have trouble conceiving babies due to blocked Fallopian tubes, thus making endometriosis a leading cause of infertility.

Symptoms are the first real clue to diagnosis. Diagnosis also involves a pelvic exam just before the menstrual period since this is the easiest time to locate areas of endometriosis. When the diagnosis is obscure — as it often is during the early stages — visual inspection of the pelvic cavity with laparoscopy may be necessary. (See Chapter 18.)

Treatment depends on your symptoms. Doctors often advise young women with symptoms of early endometriosis to become pregnant as soon as possible. Areas of endometriosis rapidly shrink and often disappear. (This varies, however, from woman to woman.) If pregnancy isn't desired or possible, taking high doses of hormone therapy over a period of six to twelve months is the next best thing. Like pregnancy, hormone therapy works by shrinking up bits of endometriosis. While doctors prescribe various types of hormone therapy, combination birth control pills are currently the most popular. Yet a new type of hormone therapy, danazol (Danocrine), may challenge their popularity. While both types of therapy essentially work by preventing ovulation and menstrual periods, danazol definitely seems to be more effective. Whether or not danazol will replace the combination pills entirely remains to be seen. Until all the results of ongoing clinical studies are in, danazol is only being used in selected cases.

Sometimes damage to the pelvic organs is so great, however, that no amount of medication helps. Here surgery is necessary. For a woman who wants to maintain her reproductive ability, bits of endometriosis can be removed from the ovaries, Fallopian tubes, uterus, and any other affected organs. If the uterus is tied down, it can be freed up and resuspended in a normal position. Temporary hormone therapy after surgery is often necessary to prevent future flare-ups. Yet, the success of this type of surgery varies greatly from woman to woman. In some women, hysterectomy may be the only way to cure severe endometriosis.

☐ FIBROIDS

Fibroids—also known as myomas or leiomyomas—are very common. In fact, about one out of five women between the ages of 30 and 45 eventually gets fibroids or noncancerous growths of the uterus. Nobody really knows what causes fibroids. Yet the ovarian hormone estrogen seems to play a role in their growth. This appears to be why fibroids continue to develop and grow in menstruating women, especially black women. On the contrary, fibroids stop growing and often shrink during the menopausal years when the ovaries stop producing estrogens.

Consisting of muscle and fibrous tissue, fibroids can vary tremendously in number, size, and location. Though it is possible to have just one fibroid, it is much more common to have several located throughout the uterus. Beginning as small, hard seedlings, fibroids can slowly grow to the size of a pea or — in rare situations — larger than a grapefruit. Even so, most fibroids remain small. Moreover, they can take up any of several locations in the uterus: in the thick muscular wall; inside the cavity; or on the outer surface of the uterus.

Depending on their size and location, fibroids may or may not cause symptoms. Usually fibroids are too small to cause symptoms. Some, however, can cause bleeding between menstrual periods in addition to longer, heavier, and more painful periods. Also, fibroids — if they become large enough — can press against the bladder (causes the need to urinate frequently) or against the bowels (causes constipation). As a rule, fibroids don't interfere with fertility or pregnancy. However, if they block the Fallopian tubes, pregnancy can be very difficult. Moreover, fibroids that bulge into the uterus during pregnancy can cause miscarriages and premature births. In women who carry their babies to term, cesarean section may be necessary if fibroids block the birth canal.

If you develop any of these symptoms, consult a doctor for a medical diagnosis. Diagnosis involves a pelvic exam to locate any fibroids. The next step is a D and C. (See Chapter 18.) If the D and C is inconclusive, visual inspection of the pelvic cavity with laparoscopy may be necessary. If there is still doubt, laparotomy — surgical exploration of the pelvic cavity — may be needed to confirm the diagnosis of fibroids. (See Chapter 18, Laparotomy and Laparoscopy.)

Treatment depends on your symptoms and the problems they may be causing. Since many fibroids are small — and don't usually cause symptoms — many doctors advise regular gynecologic exams every six months. These exams are necessary to keep track of any changes in the size and shape of the fibroids. Since fibroids tend to stop growing and shrink after the menopause, this medical approach is very practical for a great many women. If fibroids become painful and troublesome, hysterectomy is often the treatment of choice. (If your fibroids don't cause symptoms but your doctor recommends a hysterectomy, get a second surgical opinion.)

For women with symptoms who want to have more children, it *may* be possible to have the fibroids removed with myomectomy. This surgical procedure removes only the fibroids and leaves the uterus. But myomectomy is not without problems. Though the uterus is not removed, the amount of bleeding at surgery (in addition to postoperative complications) may be as high — or even higher — for myomectomy as for hysterectomy. Moreover, if the thick muscular wall of the uterus needs to be opened, future deliveries usually require cesarean section. In addition, fibroids recur in about one out of three women after myomectomy, particularly in women younger than age 45. When this happens, hysterectomy — rather than another myomectomy — is often necessary.

☐ OVARIAN CYSTS

Every year thousands of women are told, "You have an enlarged ovary." Regardless of how frightening this may sound, during the menstruating years it is most likely to be an ovarian cyst.

There are many different types of cysts which form in the ovary. But the most common type develops when an ovarian follicle grows large during ovulation. Here is how this can happen. Normally, one of the ovaries ripens a follicle each month and matures the egg it contains. When the egg matures, it leaves the follicle and escapes from the ovary (ovulation). Under normal situations, the follicle collapses and disappears after the egg leaves it. Sometimes, for unknown reasons, the follicle does not disappear. Instead, it enlarges on the surface of the ovary, fills with clear fluid, and develops into a "follicle cyst."

Most follicle cysts, which rarely get bigger than the size of a lemon, seldom cause problems. In fact, most women are unaware of having a cyst until their doctor discovers one during a routine pelvic exam. Usually follicle cysts don't require treatment, since they frequently disappear spontaneously after one or two menstrual cycles. For this reason, most doctors advise a repeat pelvic exam within two to three months to keep track of any change in the size of the cyst.

There are many other types of cysts. Some may cause dull, aching abdominal pain, particularly during the menstrual period. Heavy, irregular, and missed periods can also be symptoms. Some ovarian cysts can actually grow to be quite large — the size of a basketball and even larger — before producing any symptoms.

The best protection against ovarian cysts is to have regular pelvic exams. If you develop *any* type of cyst that does not disappear after one to two menstrual cycles, increases in size, and/or starts to cause pain or other symptoms, surgery is necessary. Diagnosis requires visual inspection of the pelvic cavity with laparoscopy or laparotomy. (See Chapter 18.) If the cyst requires removal, your doctor can usually remove it, while leaving the ovary. Fortunately, very few ovarian cysts are cancerous. Those that are require hysterectomy with removal of both Fallopian tubes and ovaries.

☐ **PELVIC INFLAMMATORY DISEASE**

Pelvic inflammatory disease — infection of the uterus, Fallopian tubes, ovaries, and/or pelvic cavity — can have any number of causes. For instance, if you use an intrauterine device, or get gonorrhea, the chances of getting this infection are high. Infection after abortion — due to incomplete abortion or unsterilized instruments, for example — is another common cause. And there are others.

The newest addition to this list is the intrauterine device

(IUD). While this fact has been known for several years, the Food and Drug Administration recently issued new, stronger warnings. This is because recent studies show that the risk of infection from IUDs is even greater than previously thought. It turns out that IUD users are three to five times more likely than nonusers to develop this infection. According to the Food and Drug Administration, IUD users at high risk for getting pelvic inflammatory disease include: women with a history of this infection; women under age 25 who have never delivered a baby; and women with more than one sex partner. In addition, IUD users who get gonorrhea are at especially high-risk for developing pelvic inflammatory disease. Despite these findings, the IUD is still considered a safe and highly effective method of birth control: still safer than the Pill. But if you want to use the IUD, be sure to receive the drug manufacturer's brochure that explains the risks and benefits of the IUD.

The first sign of pelvic inflammatory disease is usually a change in the menstrual period. Periods may begin too soon, last longer than usual, or be especially heavy. Moreover, abdominal cramping may be severe. The real trouble begins when the infection spreads from the uterus to the Fallopian tubes, causing inflammation and the development of pus within the tubal passageways (salpingitis). From the tubes, the infection can then spread to the ovaries and into the pelvic cavity (peritonitis).

If early symptoms were minimal, ignored, or even absent, once this infection gets past the uterus it usually produces real distress. Lower abdominal pain during or after the menstrual period, an obvious discharge, fever, chills, and occasionally vomiting are among the common symptoms. See a doctor promptly if you develop any of these symptoms. A delay of a day or two may well make the difference between complete recovery and permanent tubal damage.

Reports show that about 15 percent to 25 percent of all women become sterile as a result of tubal scarring and blockage from only one attack of pelvic inflammatory disease. Another disturbing aspect of this problem is its tendency to flare-up or recur after treatment. With each additional attack, the risk of becoming sterile increases. Not only that: if an egg from the ovary enters a scarred tube and becomes fertilized, pregnancy can develop in the tube instead of the uterus. Such pregnancies (ectopic) are dangerous since the tubes are too small to support a pregnancy. (If you miss one period and develop other signs of pregnancy, go to a doctor for a pregnancy test.) Lastly, women with pelvic inflammatory disease who develop a pregnancy in the uterus experience high rates of miscarriage, premature births, and stillbirths.

Early diagnosis and treatment may well make the difference between complete recovery and infertility. Treatment varies with the degree of infection. Mild forms usually require only antibiotics and bedrest at home, sometimes in the hospital. Certain severe or recurrent cases of pelvic inflammatory disease often require hysterectomy. This is because pelvic inflammatory disease can be life-threatening.

If you develop pelvic inflammatory disease while using an IUD, it may be necessary to have it removed. If you become pregnant with an IUD in place, go to a doctor promptly. The Food and Drug Administration advises doctors to remove *all* IUDs in pregnant women. It turns out that when pregnancy continues with an IUD in place, chances are high it will cause a miscarriage, which may be accompanied by infection (septic abortion).

☐ **POLYPS**

Polyps — small, red, tear-shaped growths that usually dangle on a stalk — can arise in the cervix or lining of the uterus. Cervical polyps, generally the result of a cervical infection, develop in the cervical canal. The other type, endometrial polyps, sprouts from the lining of the uterus. Common among menopausal women, endometrial polyps represent an overgrowth of normal tissue in the lining of the uterus.

Often polyps don't cause symptoms. In fact, many women are unaware of having polyps until their doctor discovers one at a routine pelvic exam. When they do cause trouble, it is usually spotting or bleeding between menstrual periods, after douching or sexual intercourse.

Medical diagnosis, which often serves as treatment, involves tissue scrapings from the uterus and cervical canal. (See Chapter 18, D and C.) Sometimes, polyps can be removed — with little discomfort — in the doctor's office. Rarely, after microscopic examination, are polyps cancerous. When they are, hysterectomy is usually necessary.

☐ URINARY STRESS INCONTINENCE

Under the slightest physical stress — a sneeze, cough, laugh, lifting, or walking, for example — certain women suddenly and involuntarily lose some urine. Varying in amount from a few drops to a puddle, urinary stress incontinence is perhaps one of the most common and distressing urologic problems among women. Usually caused by relaxation of the muscles around the bladder neck and urethra, it often occurs — at least to some degree — in women who have delivered several babies. But some women who have never been pregnant also develop this condition from time to time. While stress incontinence may start during the reproductive years, it tends to become worse over time after the menopause.

If you develop this problem, see a doctor for diagnosis and treatment since vaginal and bladder infections can cause similar symptoms. Mild stress incontinence can be helped with Kegel exercises. To do them, voluntarily tighten up the muscles you use to avoid urinating. To practice, try to start and stop your urine. (Ask your doctor how often to do these exercises.) Surgery may eventually be necessary to reposition the urethra if stress incontinence becomes severe. Success with surgery, however, varies from woman to woman and is not always curative. Practical yet temporary ways of dealing with this problem include keeping your bladder empty by frequent urination, cutting back on coffee and tea, and wearing frequently-changed minipads to minimize odor problems.

6

BIRTH CONTROL: AN OVERVIEW

☐ PREGNANCY AND PREVENTION

Whether and when to have children is up to you. Since hope and having sex just once in a while won't prevent pregnancy, most men and women use some method of birth control to:

Avoid pregnancy outside of marriage.
Avoid or postpone pregnancy for health, professional, financial, emotional, or other personal reasons.
Limit family size for such reasons as health, finances, career, and population control.

Why is birth control necessary? Because, during sexual intercourse, the man ejaculates about 400 million sperm from his penis into the woman's vagina. Resembling tadpoles, sperm speed — if uninterrupted by any method of birth control — through the vagina, cervix, and uterus. In less than one hour, about two thousand sperm reach the Fallopian tubes. If an egg is present in one of the tubes and conditions are favorable, one sperm unites with an egg — a process called "conception." Over the next several days, the fertilized egg travels down the tube to the uterus where it implants itself in the lining of the uterus. After fertilization — if conditions are favorable — the fetus develops in the uterus during the nine months of pregnancy.

Conception: union of a sperm and an egg

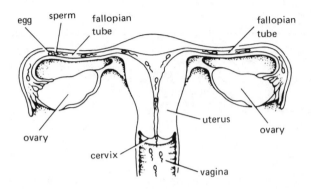

Most pregnancies occur at midcycle after one egg leaves the ovary. (See Chapter 2, Physiology of the Menstrual Cycle.) If you have unprotected sexual intercourse before ovulation, your partner's sperm can live up to five days in your tubes waiting for an egg. After your ovulate, the sperm and egg must unite within 12 to 24 hours after ovulation. After this time the egg cannot be fertilized.

Although many women ovulate about day 14 of their menstrual cycle, time of ovulation varies. For example, some women ovulate on day six or earlier, a few on day seventeen or later. This means that pregnancy can occur at almost *any* time of the menstrual cycle, depending on your day of ovulation.

Although it is possible that you may not become pregnant on the first, second, or even third month of unprotected sexual intercourse, about 80 percent to 90 percent of all women become pregnant within one year without using any method of birth control. For this reason, if you want to avoid pregnancy, consider choosing a method of birth control suitable to your personal needs. Only by choosing a method that you and your partner like enough to use *regularly*, will you get the most protection against pregnancy.

☐ CHOOSING A METHOD OF BIRTH CONTROL

Birth control is a complicated and controversial subject. This is not surprising when you consider that:

> There is currently no ideal method of birth control for everyone.
>
> The easiest and most effective methods have a wide array of minor and major side effects.
>
> Many women cannot tolerate or use the highly-effective methods.
>
> Methods with the fewest side effects are inconvenient and less effective.
>
> Depending on your needs, you will probably change your method of birth control several times throughout your reproductive years.

Currently a wide range of methods exists. Anyone can obtain some of these without a doctor's prescription or advice. Others require a prescription and medical consultation. How, then, can you choose a method that is best for you? Choice depends upon a variety of factors, and what is good for one person may not be advisable for another. Before making a decision to use any method of birth control there are several factors to consider. Ask yourself if the method is:

> Safe enough?
> Effective enough?
> Convenient and easy-to-use?
> Inexpensive enough?
> Suitable to your personal needs and lifestyle?

Then evaluate your needs:

> How much do you want to avoid pregnancy?
> How do you feel about using abortion if your method fails?
> How often do you engage in intercourse?

Are you unable to use certain methods for medical or religious reasons?

Do you mind if your method requires touching your genitals?

Do you mind if your method requires preparation at the time of intercourse?

How much access do you have to medical care?

Safety and effectiveness are the first things to consider when choosing a method of birth control. For example, women using the birth control pill may pay a price for its high level of effectiveness and convenience. (Ask a doctor about your health risks.) At the same end of the spectrum is effectiveness. Any method used exactly according to directions will have a very high level of "theoretical" effectiveness. On the other hand, most of us are careless from time to time. We may forget to take a Pill; we may remove the diaphragm too soon; or forget to insert extra vaginal spermicide with every act of intercourse. After you consider human errors such as these, you have the "use" effectiveness of any method. Unfortunately, drug manufacturers, doctors, and clinics often only refer to the theoretical effectiveness of the various methods. So be sure to ask about both the theoretical *and* use effectiveness of any method you want to use. (See Table 3.)

All methods are evaluated on their ability to prevent pregnancy based on "100 women years." For example, this

TABLE 3. Effectiveness of Birth Control Methods

METHODS	THEORETICAL EFFECTIVENESS (%)	USE EFFECTIVENESS (%)
Sterilization	99–100	99–100
Oral contraceptive	99	96
Intrauterine device	98	95
Condom and spermicidal foam	99	95
Diaphragm	97	80–90
Condom	97	80–90
Spermicidal foam	97	75–85
Rhythm (calendar method)	85	65–85

table shows that oral contraceptives have a 96 percent use effectiveness rate which is the same as a four percent pregnancy rate. This means that if you use the Pill for one year, you have about four chances out of one hundred of becoming pregnant. This rate allows for slip-ups such as forgetting to take a Pill. By comparison, if you take your Pills exactly according to directions, this method can be 99 percent effective (theoretical effectiveness rate).

The following chapters on birth control look at effectiveness; how each method works; who can use each method; what side effects may be related to their use; plus the pros and cons of each method. Compare the different methods and choose one with the help of your own doctor, local Planned Parenthood Center, public health department, or hospital birth control clinic. Next, learn how to use your method correctly and regularly. Only then can any of these methods be put to good use.

7

ORAL CONTRACEPTIVES (THE PILL)

No one calls them oral contraceptives or birth control pills anymore. It's the Pill. And more U.S. women go on the Pill than any other method because it works so well and it is such a carefree method of birth control. This trend has been going on since the Food and Drug Administration approved its use in 1960. Right now estimates show that about 10 to 15 million American women use the Pill. Worldwide, there are about 55 million users.

Despite these statistics, many women do not know how these hormones work and what they can do. From the start, the Pill has been a subject of controversy. While many doctors feel the Pill is far safer statistically than pregnancy, others rarely prescribe it; even though it is considered safe for most women. But careful research studies show that the Pill is not for all women. A few Pill users run into serious trouble.

Whether or not you can use the Pill is based on your medical history and a gynecologic physical exam. (See Table 4.) Before your doctor gives you a prescription for the Pill, ask about its risks and benefits. Along with your prescription be sure to get a brochure which explains the Pill in detail. Because of a 1976 ruling by the Food and Drug Administration (FDA), drug manufacturers now provide patient brochures with all birth control pill prescriptions. This brochure explains how the Pill works, who can use it, what side effects it may have, and what health problems may be related to

TABLE 4. Contraindications: Who Should Not Use the Pill

Certain women should not use the Pill since it may produce serious complications. Others may be able to do so under close medical supervision only. Whether you can use the Pill is based on your medical history and a gynecologic physical exam. Check this list to see if you have a medical history of any of the following conditions.

WHO SHOULD NOT USE THE PILL

Blood clots in the legs, lungs, or elsewhere in the body
Heart attack or stroke
Chest pain on exertion (angina pectoris)
Liver disease
Cancer of the breast or reproductive system
Unusual vaginal bleeding that has not been diagnosed by a doctor
Known or suspected pregnancy
Scanty or irregular menstrual periods
Young women without regular menstrual cycles
Women over 35–40
Heavy smokers (more than 15 cigarettes a day)

WHO MAY BE ABLE TO USE THE PILL UNDER CLOSE MEDICAL SUPERVISION ONLY

Strong family history of breast cancer
Benign breast disease (fibrocystic disease, breast lumps, or an abnormal
  mammogram)
Suspicious or abnormal Pap test
DES-exposed daughters
Breast-feeding
Diabetes
High blood pressure
High blood cholesterol
Migraine headaches
Kidney disease
Heart disease
Asthma
Problems during a prior pregnancy
Epilepsy
Depression
Fibroids of the uterus
Gallbladder disease
Sickle-cell disease
Varicose veins
Elective surgery planned in next four weeks

its use. Read it carefully and consult your doctor or birth control specialist if you have any questions.

While taking the Pill, you need to have a checkup every six to twelve months. (See Chapter 1, Health Care Checkups.) Be sure to have your blood pressure checked every six months or so, since it is widely known that the Pill can cause high blood pressure in some women.

If you develop problems between visits, call your doctor promptly. It may be necessary for you to change to a different Pill or stop the Pill altogether. And, if you plan to stay on the Pill, remember to schedule your return appointment before your prescription runs out.

☐ EFFECTIVENESS

Theoretical Effectiveness

Used exactly according to directions, the Pill can be 99 percent effective.

Use Effectiveness

Allowing for slip-ups (such as forgetting to take a Pill), the Pill is about 96 percent effective, which is the same as a four percent pregnancy rate. This means that if you use the Pill for one year, you have four chances out of one hundred of becoming pregnant.

☐ TYPES

Since Pills first became available, a wide array of Pills have flooded the market, while others have been taken off. Currently there are two types of Pills which require a doctor's prescription and close medical supervision: combinations and minipills. Doctors prescribe combinations far more frequently than minipills. This is because combinations are more effective in preventing pregnancy and have fewer annoying side effects than minipills.

In 1976 the FDA urged drug manufacturers to withdraw sequentials, a third type of birth control pill, from U.S. and Canadian markets. This advice became necessary when 1975 case reports suggested an association between cancer of the endometrium (lining of the uterus) and use of sequential pills. A 1976 research study, later confirmed by other studies, also suggested an association between endometrial hyperplasia and long-term use of sequentials. Hyperplasia is the term that describes an overgrowth of cells of the endometrium. Occasionally, certain types of hyperplasia may change to very early cancer (also called cancer *in situ*) and eventually to invasive cancer.

Sequentials were different in hormonal composition than combinations. They contained high doses of estrogens alone for most of the cycle plus progestin as well as estrogens for five days at the end of the cycle. But doctors did not routinely prescribe sequentials (Oracon, Ortho Novum Sq., and Norquin). In fact, they were an alternative to combinations for women who required higher doses of estrogens. Only five to ten percent of all women received sequentials for special problems such as late first menstrual period, very irregular periods, and acne.

Combinations

In 1960 the FDA approved the use of the first birth control pill, the combinations. Doctors currently prescribe them far more frequently than minipills. By and large, they are more effective in preventing pregnancy and have fewer annoying side effects. Combinations prevent pregnancy in several ways. Each monthly pack of Pills not only keeps the ovaries from releasing an egg, but it also alters the lining of the uterus and cervical mucus, making implantation of an egg highly unlikely.

What makes combinations work are two chemicals basically the same as your body's own hormones, estrogen and progesterone. Each Pill currently contains 0.3 to 10 mg of progestin and 20 to 100 mcg of estrogen. In view of 1970 research findings, most doctors now prescribe combinations containing 50 mcg of estrogen or less. (See Table 5.) A British report, later confirmed by other studies, shows that women using higher doses of estrogen are at greater risk for developing blood clots than women using Pills with 50 mcg of estrogen or less. (More about that later.)

Since 1973 several Pills containing less than 50 mcg of estrogen ("low-dose" Pills) have come on the market. In general, doctors prescribe these Pills to women requiring lower doses of estrogen. Even so, many women become discouraged when using low-dose Pills because of irregular bleeding in addition to higher pregnancy rates.

There has always been much discussion among doctors about how to choose the right Pill for each woman. But there *is* no right Pill for all women. For this reason, only take your own Pills: the ones prescribed for you. The hormone dose in a friend's prescription may be more or less than you should have. Choice of a Pill varies from woman to woman. The best Pill provides the smallest dose of hormones

---

TABLE 5. Currently Available Combination Oral Contraceptives

	AMOUNT OF ESTROGEN	
Less than 50 mcg	*50 mcg*	*More than 50 mcg*
Brevicon	Demulen	Enovid-E
Loestrin 1/20	Norlestrin 1/50	Enovid 5
Loestrin 1.5/30	Norlestrin 2.5/50	Norinyl 1+80
Lo/Ovral	Norinyl 1+50	Norinyl 2
Modicon	Ortho-Novum 1/50	Ortho-Novum 1/80
Ovcon-35	Ovcon-50	Ortho-Novum 2
Zorane 1/20	Ovral	Ortho-Novum 10
Zorane 1.5/30	Zorane 1/50	Ovulen

that will prevent pregnancy and have minimal side effects. Most doctors and clinics now *start* women on combinations containing 50 mcg of estrogen. If irregular bleeding occurs, it may be necessary to switch to a combination containing more than 50 mcg of estrogen. If so, your doctor should inform you of the risks of using a Pill with more than 50 mcg of estrogen.

Minipills

In 1973 the FDA approved use of the minipill. Doctors now prescribe the minipill far less frequently than combinations. It turns out that they are slightly less effective in preventing pregnancy and when pregnancy does occur it is more likely to be outside the uterus (ectopic). Also, minipills often cause unexpected bleeding and irregular menstrual cycles. Unlike combinations, minipills don't contain estrogen. Instead they contain .35 mg or less of progestin only. Currently available minipills include: Micronor, Nor-Q-D., and Ovrette.

How minipills prevent pregnancy is not well understood. Their effectiveness seems to depend on several factors: prevention of ovulation in some cycles; prevention of an egg from traveling through the Fallopian tube after ovulation occurs; and changes in the lining of the uterus and cervical mucus, making implantation of a fertilized egg highly unlikely.

Unfortunately, the minipill has not lived up to the expectations of those who thought it would replace the combination. Using the lowest effective hormone dose seemed wise, yet instead of replacing the combination, the minipill has become an alternative to it for women who cannot use estrogens for health reasons. Breast-feeding women who want oral contraception can also use the minipill. Unlike estrogen-containing Pills, minipills do not reduce milk production. And women unable to tolerate the estrogen-related side effects of combinations sometimes switch to the minipill.

☐ HOW TO USE

Your doctor or birth control specialist should tell you how to use your Pills. Be sure to ask questions if you don't understand. Here are some points which generally apply:

First Cycle

Most *combinations* require you to start the first Pill on day five of the menstrual cycle. (Day one is the first day of menstrual bleeding.) Some combinations are to be started on the first Sunday after the menstrual period begins. *Minipills* should be started on the first day of menstrual bleeding. If you have just delivered a baby (especially if you plan to breast-feed) or have had an abortion, ask your doctor when to start the first cycle of Pills. To be on the safe side, use a second method of contraception (such as foam and condom) during the first month of Pill use.

When to Take

Take one Pill every day, at about the same time each day. By doing this you are much less likely to forget to take a Pill. Whether or not the Pill works depends primarily on whether you faithfully take your Pill every day. (If you don't take your Pills regularly, you may ovulate and become pregnant.) You can minimize side effects, such as nausea, by taking your Pill at bedtime or with your evening meal instead of in the morning.

Most *combinations* come in packs of 21 hormone Pills. Take one Pill every day for 21 days; stop for seven days. Bleeding begins in several days. Start a new pack of Pills on day eight, even if you are still bleeding or have not gotten your period. A few combinations come in packs of 28 Pills (21 hormone and 7 without hormone). Take these Pills every day of the year. Bleeding begins while taking the seven non-hormone Pills. The 28-day pack of Pills is good for women who don't want the bother of an off-and-on schedule of Pill taking.

The *minipills* come in packs of 28 hormone Pills. Take these every day of the year, even during bleeding.

Forgotten Pills

If you forget *one* Pill, take the forgotten Pill as soon as you remember and take the next Pill at the regular time. If you forget *two* Pills, take two Pills as soon as you remember and take two Pills the next day. Use an additional method of contraception for the rest of your cycle. If you forget *three* or more Pills, you will probably ovulate, menstrual bleeding (more properly called "withdrawal bleeding") will begin, and pregnancy can occur. Start using another method of contraception immediately. Throw out the old pack of Pills and start a new pack seven days after you took the last Pill, even if you are still bleeding. Use a second method of contraception for the first month of using your new pack of Pills.

Skipped Menstrual Periods

If you forget *one* or more Pills and skip *one* menstrual period, arrange a pregnancy test with your doctor or clinic. If you didn't forget any Pills, but you do skip *one* period, the chances of pregnancy are slim. It is common for Pill users, especially minipill users, to skip periods occasionally. If you didn't forget any Pills but skip *two* periods, arrange a pregnancy test.

Going Off the Pill

If you stop taking the Pill, you can become pregnant the next month. If you do not want to become pregnant, use another method of birth control. But if you are planning a pregnancy, use another method of contraception for at least three months before trying to conceive. This will help insure a healthy pregnancy.

□ SIDE EFFECTS AND COMPLICATIONS

Over the past 15 years or so many women have taken the Pill, with an excellent track record of safety and satisfaction. Yet the Pill is known to cause certain side effects and complications. (See Table 6.) In general, these are hormone-related and dose-related. Some are common and not serious, while others are rare and may be life-threatening. Though it is considered safe for most women, careful studies show that the Pill is not for all women. Lots of women don't notice any side effects, except for mild passing ones. But a few Pill users run into serious trouble. Whether or not the Pill is for you is based on your medical history and a gynecologic physical exam (with blood pressure measurement). If you develop any kind of side effect, call your doctor promptly.

Common and Less Common Side Effects

These side effects can be divided into two groups: those that mimic pregnancy and those that are directly related to the menstrual cycle. The symptoms of pseudopregnancy that are usually estrogen-related include: fluid retention; headaches; nausea or vomiting; urinary tract infection; vaginal discharge and infection; tender or enlarged breasts; and spotty darkening of the skin, especially of the face. These symptoms frequently occur among users of the combination Pill. With the exception of nausea, these symptoms may also occur among minipill users. Other symptoms of pseudopregnancy that are usually progestin-related include: weight gain; acne; depression, mood changes, fatigue; and a decrease in sexual desire and response. These symptoms occur in users of the combination and less frequently in users of the minipill.

TABLE 6. Side Effects and Complications of the Pill

| SIDE EFFECTS | TIME OF SIDE EFFECT | | |
	Worse in First 3 Months	Constant	Worse Over Time
MOST COMMON			
Fluid retention	*		
Headaches		*	
Nausea and vomiting	*		
Urinary tract infection			*
Vaginal discharge and infection			*
Weight gain	*		
LESS COMMON			
Acne		*	
Bleeding or spotting between periods	*		
Breast tenderness and fullness	*		
Change in cycle (flow and length)		*	
Decrease in sexual desire and response		*	
Depression, mood changes, fatigue		*	
Missed periods			*
Spotty darkening of skin, especially on face			*
Worsening of pre-existing conditions: migraine, asthma, epilepsy, fibroids of uterus, and kidney or heart disease		*	
RARE			
Blood clots to brain, legs, and lungs		*	
Gallbladder disease			*
Heart attack			*
High blood pressure			*
Noncancerous liver tumors			*

In addition to the symptoms of pseudopregnancy, most Pill users experience some change in their menstrual cycle. On the whole, women using combinations experience more regular cycles that are shorter in length with lighter bleeding. Combinations also lessen abdominal discomfort, crampiness, and the symptoms of premenstrual tension. The "low-dose" combinations — with their low level of estrogen — tend to produce irregular bleeding between periods. Common problems of the minipill include: unexpected bleeding between periods, irregular cycles, and missed periods.

The Pill can also aggravate or worsen conditions such as: depression, migraine, asthma, epilepsy, fibroids of the uterus, kidney disease, and heart disease. If you have one of these conditions, you *may* be able to use the Pill under close medical supervision only. If your condition becomes worse while using the Pill, contact your doctor promptly.

Unless your symptoms are severe, doctors advise women to stay on the Pill since it takes time for the body to adjust to these new hormone levels. In the end, this is usually better than shifting from one Pill to the next. If your side effects don't go away on their own, switching to Pills with a different estrogen/progestin mix often helps.

Rare Side Effects

The following side effects are rare. Few Pill users ever run into serious trouble. If you develop any of these problems, stop taking the Pill, call your doctor promptly, and choose another method of contraception.

Blood Clots. The first side effect found to be associated with the Pill was blood clotting disease (thrombophlebitis). Since the first case reports in the early 1960s, British and U.S. research studies have shown that Pill users are five to ten times more likely than non-Pill users to develop blood clots. So far minipill users do not appear to be "at risk." These blood clots have occurred primarily in the legs and less frequently in the brain and heart. Every year, about one woman out of every two thousand Pill users is hospitalized for blood clots, mostly for clots in the leg. Blood clots that remain in the leg (phlebitis) are relatively common and are usually not dangerous. Clots that travel to the lungs (pulmonary embolism), or form in the brain (stroke), or heart are rare. They can, on rare occasions, be extremely serious and cause death.

The British and U.S. data show that the effect of the Pill varies with the type of blood clot, estrogen dose, age, and smoking habits. Though risk estimates from these studies do vary, the frequently-quoted British studies report that:

> *Leg (phlebitis)*: Pill users are about 2.4 times more likely than non-Pill users to develop phlebitis.
>
> *Leg (vein thrombosis)*: Pill users are about 4.2 times more likely than non-Pill users to develop vein thrombosis.
>
> *Pulmonary embolism.* Pill users are about 2.4 times more likely than non-Pill users to develop a pulmonary embolism.
>
> *Brain (stroke)*: Pill users are about 4 times more likely than non-Pill users to develop a stroke.

The data also show that the risk of developing blood clots varies with estrogen dose. Since 1970 studies have revealed that women using high dose Pills are at greater risk than women using Pills with 50 mcg of estrogen or less. (See Table 5.) In view of the 1970 recommendations from the British Committee on Safety and Drugs and the U.S. Food and Drug Administration, most doctors now prescribe Pills containing 50 mcg of estrogen or less.

Other factors are also involved. The risk of developing clots begins at age 30, especially for heavy smokers (15 or more cigarettes a day). The older you get, the higher the risk. Over age 35, the risk is very serious: either quit smoking or consider another method of contraception. Over age 40, the Pill is out, whether you smoke or not.

Right now it does not appear that the risk of developing clots is related to how long you use the Pill. Also, once you stop the Pill you do not remain at any higher risk for developing clots than non-Pill users.

If you develop trouble while using the Pill, call your doctor promptly. Serious problems hardly ever occur without warning. Some Pill users experience symptoms (which should not be ignored) for weeks or months before seeking medical attention. Signs of trouble, possibly serious trouble, may include:

> Chest pain or shortness of breath.
> Coughing up blood.
> Severe headache or vomiting.
> Severe pain in the leg or arm.
> Dizziness or fainting.
> Blurred vision, loss of vision, or flashing lights.

If you develop any of these symptoms, go to your doctor or hospital emergency room immediately.

Heart Attack. Since 1975 several studies have strongly suggested that estrogen Pill users are at higher risk for developing heart attacks than non-Pill users. Of great significance is that risk increases with age: Pill users over age 35 are at higher risk than Pill users under age 35. In view of these findings, if you are over age 35 and have one or more risk factors for a heart attack — 15 or more cigarettes a day; diabetes; obesity; hypertension; or high amount of fats in the blood stream — choose another method of contraception. Over age 40, the Pill is out, whether or not you have one of these risk factors.

If you develop any of the following symptoms, go to your doctor or hospital emergency room immediately. These may be signs of trouble:

> Severe chest pain or shortness of breath.
> Weakness, sweating, nausea.

High Blood Pressure. Since the 1960s numerous studies have reported an association between high blood pressure and estrogen-containing Pills. The increase in blood pressure is usually slight and reversible three to four months after stopping the Pill. Even so, the risk of developing high blood pressure does increase after several years of Pill use. In a few women, the rise in blood pressure may be severe (hypertension). Mild hypertension usually does not cause symptoms.

Symptoms of severe hypertension may develop gradually after several years of Pill use. These include: headaches; dizziness; fatigue; nervousness; insomnia; palpitations; weakness; and, possibly, nosebleeds. Call your doctor if you develop any of these symptoms. Also, be sure your six month checkup includes measurement of your blood pressure. Any exam lacking this test is incomplete.

Gallbladder Disease. Since 1973 several research studies have reported an association between the Pill and gallbladder disease (inflammation of the gallbladder and gallstones). Even though this side effect is rare, the risk of developing gallstones (cholesterol deposits in the gallbladder) increases after several years of Pill use. Gallstones are often symptom-free. Yet they may cause indigestion or severe upper abdominal pain with chills and fever — symptoms you should report to your doctor immediately.

Noncancerous Liver Tumors. Since 1972 numerous studies have shown an association between the Pill and noncancerous liver tumors. The risk is very low. Only 150 or so Pill users have developed liver tumors. Women who use estrogen Pills for longer than five years, however, appear to be at much higher risk than women who use the Pill for a shorter period of time. Some of these tumors are without symptoms and complications, while others may cause abdominal fullness, pressure, or severe pain. Because some of these tumors may lead to serious complications and be fatal, be sure to report these symptoms to your doctor immediately.

Proven Or Unproven?

Studies have suggested, but not yet proven, that the Pill may be related to cancer, lack of menstrual periods after stopping the Pill, elevated levels of sugar in the blood, birth defects, and a wide array of other conditions. While there is no clear evidence that the Pill causes these problems, you should be aware of the possibility. Right now researchers are trying to determine whether the Pill actually causes these conditions or not.

Cancer. Does the Pill cause cancer or precancerous conditions, accelerate cancer growth, or can it actually reduce the risk of developing benign disease? Numerous research studies have tried to evaluate whether the Pill has a cancer-causing effect on the breasts and reproductive system. Current findings do not show any relationship between cancer and use of the combination or minipill. In 1969 a research study suggested that Pill users are at greater risk than nonusers for developing precancerous conditions of the cervix. Many studies challenged these findings. Now it is generally agreed that there is no firm evidence that the Pill causes these conditions. Yet many epidemiologists feel that additional time — perhaps as long as 10 to 20 years — may be needed to observe whether the Pill can have a cancer-causing effect.

In 1976 the Food and Drug Administration urged drug manufacturers to withdraw sequentials, a third type of birth control pill, from U.S. and Canadian markets. This advice became necessary when 1975 case reports suggested an association between endometrial cancer and use of sequential pills. A 1976 research study, later confirmed by other studies, also suggested an association between endometrial hyperplasia and long-term use of sequentials. Hyperplasia is the term that describes an overgrowth of cells in the endometrium. Occasionally certain types of hyperplasia may change to very early cancer (also called cancer *in situ*) and eventually to invasive cancer. Sequentials were different in hormonal composition than combinations and minipills. They contained high doses of estrogens alone for most of the cycle plus progestin as well as estrogens for five days at the end of the cycle.

Since 1970 numerous studies have reported that the Pill does not increase but actually reduces the risk of developing certain types of benign breast disease. It is well known that women with a history of certain types of benign breast disease are at higher risk for developing breast cancer. Even so, there is no evidence that the Pill offers protection against breast cancer, though it protects against the development of benign breast disease. Further time may be needed to observe what relationship (if any) exists between breast cancer and the Pill.

Right now doctors advise women with a history of cancer of the breast or reproductive system not to use the Pill. Moreover, if you have a medical history of any of the following conditions, you *may* be able to use the Pill under close medical supervision only: women with a strong family history of breast cancer; women with fibrocystic disease, breast lumps, or an abnormal mammogram; and women with a suspicious or abnormal Pap test.

Post-Pill Lack of Menstrual Periods. Lack of menstrual periods (secondary amenorrhea) after stopping the Pill is becoming a common problem. Whether or not the Pill is responsible is uncertain. In general, women more likely to develop this problem include those with irregular menstrual cycles before starting the Pill and young women who started to menstruate late (16 years or older). Most women resume their periods several months after stopping the Pill. If you don't get your menstrual period within six months, see your doctor.

Lack of periods can also be a sign of pregnancy. If you develop symptoms of pregnancy — nausea, or vomiting, need to urinate more often, tender breasts, need to sleep more than usual — arrange a pregnancy test with your doctor or clinic.

Elevated Levels of Sugar in the Blood. In the mid-1960s several studies noted changes in sugar and insulin metabolism in a group of Pill users with the "glucose tolerance" laboratory test. While this change may occur, it is reversible several months after stopping the Pill. Pill users at higher risk for developing this condition include women with: early undetected diabetes; a family history of diabetes; and obesity. Even though diabetic Pill users may be bothered by this problem, pregnancy presents even greater hazards. If you are diabetic and want to use the Pill, you need to have regular medical checkups while using the Pill. As for nondiabetic women, there is no evidence that the Pill increases the risk of developing diabetes, during or after using the Pill.

Birth Defects. Since 1973 several studies have suggested that women taking estrogen and/or progestin during the first three months of pregnancy may be at greater risk for bearing babies with birth defects. This possibility is particularly linked to the hormone progestin. These infant abnormalities include: the absence of all or part of arms, legs, fingers, toes, in addition to organ defects, especially heart. Various types of hormonal exposures have been implicated: first, as a pregnancy test; secondly, as therapy for the high-risk pregnancy; and thirdly, accidentally taking the Pill early in pregnancy.

Because of a 1977 ruling by the Food and Drug Administration, drug manufacturers now provide patient brochures with all prescriptions containing progestin. Right now progestin is used in the birth control pill and in drugs to treat menstrual disorders, the high-risk pregnancy, and abnormal bleeding of the uterus. Progestin is no longer used in pregnancy tests.

For your safety, make sure you are not pregnant before starting the Pill. If you think you are pregnant, use another method of contraception until your menstrual period confirms nonpregnancy. If you are planning pregnancy, use another method of birth control (such as foam and condom) for at least three months before trying to conceive to help insure a healthy pregnancy. If you become pregnant while using the Pill, consult your doctor about the risks and advisability of continuing your pregnancy.

☐ PROS AND CONS

Pros

Most effective and carefree method of birth control.
Requires no preparation at the time of intercourse.
Convenient and easy-to-use.

Produces more regular cycles, relief of premenstrual tension, and fewer menstrual cramps.

Reduces the likelihood of developing iron deficiency anemia that is common in menstruating women.

Useful for treating endometriosis.

Cons

Long list of side effects and complications. (Some are life-threatening.)

Many women cannot use the Pill.

Must remember to take one Pill every day.

Requires closer medical supervision than any other method.

Inconvenient for women who have sex infrequently.

8

INTRAUTERINE DEVICES (IUDs)

Most of them look like plastic earrings, but they are intra-uterine devices, or IUDs for short. No matter what they look like — coils, 7's, loops, or T's — they do their job well. Currently used by some three million American women, IUDs provide highly effective, inexpensive, and simple contraception. It is a method that you don't have to make work. It works by itself. And, when it comes to effectiveness in preventing pregnancy, IUDs are second only to the birth control pill.

At the same time, the IUD has its share of problems. Though considered safe for many women, the IUD is not for all women. Moreover, a few IUD users run into serious trouble. Whether you can use the IUD is based on your medical history and a gynecologic physical exam. (See Table 7.) Before the doctor inserts your IUD, be sure to ask about its risks and benefits. Also, make sure you receive a brochure that explains the IUD in detail. Because of a 1975 ruling by the Food and Drug Administration (FDA), drug manufacturers now provide patient brochures with all IUDs. This brochure explains how the IUD works, who can use it, what side effects it may have, and what health problems may be related to its use. Read it carefully and consult your doctor or birth control specialist if you have any questions.

While using the IUD, you need to have a checkup exam one menstrual period after insertion and once a year after that. If you develop problems between visits, call your doc-

---

TABLE 7. Contraindications: Who Should Not Use the IUD

Certain women should not use the IUD since it may produce serious complications. Whether you can use the IUD is based on your medical history and a gynecologic physical exam. Check this list to see if you have a medical history of any of the following conditions.

Abnormalities of the uterus
Allergy to copper (for Copper 7 and Copper T)
Anemia
Menstrual problems (severe menstrual cramps; heavy periods; bleeding between periods)
Cancer of the cervix or uterus
Fainting attacks
Heart disease or heart murmur
Infection of the cervix, vagina, or uterus
Pelvic inflammatory disease
Prior IUD use
Surgery on the uterus
Recent abortion or miscarriage
Pregnancy outside the uterus
Known or suspected pregnancy
Suspicious or abnormal Pap test
Unusual vaginal bleeding that has not been diagnosed by a doctor
Venereal disease
Wilson's disease

---

tor promptly, since it may be necessary to have your IUD replaced with another size or removed altogether.

☐ EFFECTIVENESS

Theoretical Effectiveness

Used exactly according to directions, the IUD can be 98 percent effective.

Use Effectiveness

Allowing for slip-ups (such as unknowingly having sex with a displaced IUD), this method is about 95 percent effective, which is the same as a five percent pregnancy rate. This means that if you use the IUD for one year, you have five chances out of one hundred of becoming pregnant.

During the first three months after insertion, use another method of birth control (such as foam and condom) since medical opinion varies concerning IUD effectiveness during these early months

□ **TYPES**

IUDs come in assorted shapes and sizes. Most are made of flexible plastic. But some newer ones are wrapped in copper wire or contain the hormone progesterone. Ranging in size from one-inch in width to one-and-a-half inches in length, they have nylon strings that hang into the vagina when the IUD is in place.

There are several opinions about how IUDs actually work. The most common theory is that they prevent pregnancy by altering the lining of the uterus so that a fertilized egg cannot become implanted.

Nonmedicated

Most IUDs are plastic, nonmedicated or "first generation" ones. Nonmedicated IUDs, which can remain in the uterus indefinitely, currently include the Lippes Loop and Saf-T-Coil.

Some women, especially those who have never been pregnant, have difficulties with these IUDs. In fact, women who have never been pregnant may find that their uterus pushes out the IUD because it can't tolerate the device, while others experience persistent discomfort and bleeding.

Until 1974 the Dalkon Shield was nearly as common as the Lippes Loop and Saf-T-Coil. When introduced to the market, the Shield was the first nonmedicated IUD designed for the never-pregnant woman. In 1974, however, the FDA ordered drug manufacturers to withdraw the Dalkon Shield from the market. This became necessary as a result of 1973 reports associating pregnancy and the Shield in place with infected miscarriage (septic abortion). As a result of these findings, the FDA now advises doctors to remove *any* type of IUD in women who become pregnant. This is because removing an IUD early in pregnancy prevents serious complications from developing.

Medicated

Medicated or "second generation" IUDs were first approved by the FDA in 1974. Smaller than the nonmedicated ones, they were specifically designed to make IUDs more acceptable to the woman who has never been pregnant. Most are constructed of plastic and wrapped in copper wire (Copper 7 and Copper T), but some are made of rubber and contain the hormone progesterone (Progestasert). Unlike the nonmedicated IUDs, the copper ones must be replaced every two to four years and the progesterone IUD, every year. Right now there is no evidence that the copper and progesterone released from these IUDs increases the chance of developing cervical or uterine problems.

For the woman who has never been pregnant these newer IUDs are a real improvement over the older nonmedicated ones. Side effects such as persistent discomfort, bleeding, and expulsion are not nearly as common. Without a doubt these newer IUDs are more comfortable for the woman who has never been pregnant.

☐ INSERTION AND REMOVAL

The best time to have an IUD inserted is during the last day or two of your menstrual period. This is because the cervix is softer and slightly open, which makes insertion easier; the uterus more easily accepts the IUD; and at this time there is almost no chance of pregnancy. Often IUDs are also inserted after delivery (immediately or after eight weeks) or right after abortion.

Before insertion the doctor should take a complete medical history and perform a pelvic exam to rule out pregnancy, pelvic infection, and gonorrhea. (You should *never* have an IUD inserted when you are pregnant or have gonorrhea or a pelvic infection.) What type of IUD you can use—if you can use it at all—depends on the position and size of your uterus in addition to your menstrual and pregnancy history.

IUD insertion is a simple procedure that takes only a few minutes. Being quite elastic, the IUD fits into a special inserter or thin sterile tube about the size of a drinking straw. The doctor gently pushes the tube through your cervix up into your uterus. When the inserter is in proper position,

The iud

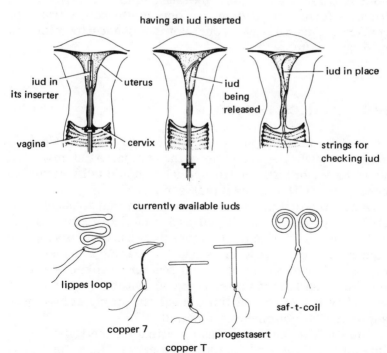

having an iud inserted

iud in its inserter | uterus | iud being released | iud in place
vagina | cervix | strings for checking iud

currently available iuds

lippes loop | copper 7 | copper T | progestasert | saf-t-coil

your doctor slowly releases the IUD out of its tube and into the uterus. After the IUD enters the uterus, it resumes its original shape.

Many women — especially women who have never been pregnant — experience some discomfort and/or pain during insertion. From time to time, some women feel lightheaded and may even faint, but this passes quickly. Some doctors routinely use local anesthesia, while others do not. Since it is much easier to prevent discomfort and cramps than to stop them, take a few aspirin beforehand to make insertion less uncomfortable.

If at any point you decide that you no longer want your IUD, a doctor can remove it. (*Never* try to remove it yourself.) As with insertion, removal is easier toward the end of the menstrual period. In most cases, fertility is restored almost immediately. If you want to become pregnant, have your IUD removed and use another method of birth control (such as foam and condom) for one month before trying to conceive. This will give your uterus a chance to return to its normal state.

□ HOW TO CHECK THE IUD

Most IUDs have nylon strings attached to them that extend down through the cervix into the vagina. After insertion, your doctor or birth control specialist should tell you how to check your IUD to make sure it is in place.

During the first month of use, it is important to check your IUD strings once a week and each time before intercourse. This is because during the first month of use there is a slightly higher rate of expulsion, especially during the menstrual period. (Remember to check all feminine napkins and tampons since an IUD can often come out without your knowing or feeling it.) After that time, check the strings at least once a month after your menstrual period.

You can check your strings by sitting on the toilet, squatting on the floor, or lying down. Insert one finger into your vagina⁻ so that you can feel your cervix. Then feel for the strings hanging down from the cervix that form the "tail" of the IUD. Sometimes the strings are hard to find, so wait a day and try again. If you still can't feel them at all or if you feel part of the IUD, it has probably slipped out of position. When this happens, call your doctor or clinic right away. In the meantime, avoid intercourse or use another method of birth control, since the IUD is not very effective when it is out of position.

□ **SIDE EFFECTS AND COMPLICATIONS**

The IUD is known to cause various side effects. (See Table 8.) With the exception of some minor annoyances during the first few months after insertion, many women don't experience difficulties. These initial reactions—though rather annoying—are the body's attempt to adapt to a foreign object in the uterus. Once in a while, though, a few IUD users

TABLE 8. Side Effects and Complications of the IUD

| SIDE EFFECTS | TIME OF SIDE EFFECT | |
	Worse in First 3 Months	Constant
COMMON		
Bleeding or spotting between periods	*	
Heavy, longer, and more crampy menstrual periods	*	
Pain (cramps and backache)	*	
Expulsion	*	
LESS COMMON		
Perforation of the uterus	*	
RARE		
Pregnancy outside the uterus		*
Septic abortion		*
Pelvic inflammatory disease		*

run into trouble. If you develop any of these problems, call your doctor promptly.

Bleeding and Pain

During the first year of use about 10 percent of all women have their IUD removed for the most common side effects, bleeding and pain. For the first few months after insertion, the menstrual cycle undergoes some changes: periods may become heavier, longer, and more crampy. There may also be some spotting or cramping between periods. If any of these symptoms becomes constant or severe, call your doctor or clinic, since prolonged bleeding can cause anemia.

Regardless of IUD type, never-pregnant women are more likely to develop bleeding and pain than women who have been pregnant.

Expulsion

While many women's bodies adapt to IUDs, some women (especially women who have never been pregnant) may find that their uterus pushes out the IUD because it can't tolerate the device. During the first few months after insertion, IUD expulsion is just about as common as bleeding and pain. At this time, the uterus either adapts to the IUD or forces it out. When this happens, the IUD usually ends up in the cervical canal or vagina. But in a few women, the IUD actually tears through the wall of the uterus and enters the abdominal cavity. (See next section.)

Perforation of the Uterus

Occasionally, IUDs can perforate or tear the uterus. Most of the time this happens during insertion. But in about one out of a thousand women the IUD actually tears through the wall of the uterus and enters the abdominal cavity. (Sometimes surgery is necessary to remove the IUD.) Since pain is sometimes — but not always — a symptom of perforation, it is essential that you regularly check your IUD to make certain it is in place.

Pregnancy

Every year about five out of a hundred women become pregnant with an IUD in place. If your menstrual period is late, see your doctor or clinic right away about a pregnancy test. If you are pregnant, the FDA advises you to have your IUD removed if the strings are visible. This is because having an IUD removed during the first three months of pregnancy decreases the likelihood of developing serious complications. When pregnancy continues with an IUD in place, chances are high it will cause a miscarriage that may be accompanied by infection (septic abortion). If at any time you develop the following symptoms, call your doctor or clinic promptly: abdominal pain or tenderness; fever; severe cramping; bleeding; or unusual vaginal discharge. These may be signs of infection.

1973 Dalkon Shield findings focused attention on the dangers of becoming pregnant with an IUD in place. The Shield was found to cause severe infection, septic abortion, and — on rare occasions — death when pregnancy continued with an IUD in place. Most of these complications occurred during the second trimester of pregnancy.

So, if you discover you are pregnant, have your IUD removed right away. At this time you and your doctor should discuss whether it is better to have an abortion or continue your pregnancy. If you choose to continue your pregnancy — whether your IUD is removed or not — the doctor should inform you of the risks of doing so.

Getting pregnant can cause other problems, too. It turns out that women who become pregnant with an IUD in place are more likely than non-IUD users to develop pregnancy outside the uterus. In fact, anywhere from three percent to nine percent of all IUD pregnancies are "ectopic" or nonuterine. Ectopic pregnancies, which usually occur in one of the Fallopian tubes, can be dangerous. After two to three months of pregnancy, the tube tears or bursts because it can no longer support a pregnancy. When this happens, surgery is necessary to stop the bleeding. Fortunately, ectopic pregnancy can often be diagnosed before this happens. So if you become pregnant while using an IUD, be sure your doctor evaluates you for the possibility of an ectopic pregnancy.

Pelvic Inflammatory Disease

Recent studies provide strong evidence that IUD users are three to five times more likely than nonusers to develop pelvic inflammatory disease. Pelvic inflammatory disease is a severe infection which starts in the uterus and can affect the Fallopian tubes, ovaries, and/or pelvic cavity. (See Chapter 5.) While this has been known for several years, the FDA recently issued new, stronger warnings. IUD users at high risk for developing this infection include: women with a history of this infection; women under age 25 who have never delivered a baby; and women with more than one sex partner. In addition, IUD users who get gonorrhea are at especially high-risk for developing pelvic inflammatory disease.

See a doctor right away if you develop any of the following symptoms: change in menstrual periods; fever; bleeding or unusual vaginal discharge; abdominal pain; or pain related to sexual intercourse. These may be signs of pelvic inflammatory disease. A delay of a day or two may well make the difference between complete recovery and infertility.

☐ **PROS AND CONS**

Pros

> Highly effective, easy-to-use method of birth control.
> Carefree method that doesn't require preparation at the time of intercourse.

With the exception of IUD cost, this method is inexpensive.

Very effective alternative for women who can't use the Pill (especially women over age 35).

Cons

See list of side effects and complications. (Some are life-threatening.) Many women stop using the IUD during the first year because of these side effects.

Many women, especially those who have never been pregnant, can't tolerate the IUD.

Must remember to check the strings to make certain the IUD is in place.

Some women don't like the idea of having an object in their uterus all the time.

Copper IUDs must be replaced every two to four years and the progesterone one every year.

9

DIAPHRAGM

Before the Pill and the IUD came along, the diaphragm was the most reliable and widely used method of birth control. Always used with spermicidal jelly or cream, this soft dome-shaped device is *still* one of the most effective methods. By covering the cervix, it blocks the passage of racing sperm in two ways: physically by the diaphragm and chemically by the spermicide. While its popularity has declined since the 1960s, women disillusioned with the health risks and side effects of the Pill and IUD have switched or returned to the diaphragm. This is because it is practically 100 percent risk-free. In more than 50 years of use in the United States, nobody has found any way the diaphragm can hurt you.

Why don't more women use the diaphragm? Most importantly, it requires a high level of motivation: it takes some patience and skill to learn how to use it. To work, it must fit correctly. This is why diaphragms are not sold over-the-counter. Your doctor or clinic must fit you, give you a prescription for the correct size, and teach you how to use it. Also, many women object to the inconvenience of having to insert it before intercourse and remove it at a later time. Other women, uncomfortable about their sexuality, feel squeamish about putting something into their vagina.

While some women may swear at the diaphragm and others swear by it, if you are searching for a safe, highly effective method of birth control, consider the diaphragm.

☐ EFFECTIVENESS

Theoretical Effectiveness

Used exactly according to directions, the diaphragm can be 97 percent effective.

Use Effectiveness

Allowing for slip-ups (such as not inserting the diaphragm correctly), this method is about 80 percent to 90 percent effective, which is the same as a 10 percent to 20 percent pregnancy rate. This means that if you use the diaphragm for one year, you have about 10 to 20 chances out of one hundred of becoming pregnant.

☐ TYPES AND THE FITTING EXAM

Diaphragms come in different sizes and styles. The diaphragm itself is a thin, soft rubber (some are plastic) cup attached to a flexible or firm metal ring. They range in size from two to four inches in diameter. The larger sizes generally fit women with one or more children while the smaller sizes are for women without children.

Four popular types of diaphragms include: the coil-spring; the flat-spring; the arching; and the bowbent.

The better a diaphragm fits, the better it stays in place during intercourse. To find out what size and type you need — or if you can use the diaphragm at all — a doctor or birth control specialist must first examine you. (See Table 9.) By inserting a series of flexible rings into your vagina, a doctor can gauge the exact size and type of diaphragm for you. A properly-fitted diaphragm not only covers the cervix, but it fits snugly and comfortably behind the pubic bone. Your body actually holds it in place. It cannot fall out unless you

TABLE 9. Contraindications: Who Should Not Use the Diaphragm

Certain women should not use the diaphragm. Whether you can use the diaphragm is based on your medical history and a gynecologic physical exam. Check this list to see if you have a medical history of any of the following conditions.

Falling of the uterus into the vagina (prolapse)
Protrusion of the bladder into the vagina (cystocele)
Protrusion of the rectum into the vagina (rectocele)
Opening in the vagina (fistula)
Severely tipped uterus
Allergy to rubber or spermicide

take it out. And you and your partner should not feel it during intercourse. On the contrary, a diaphragm that is too small moves around too much while a large one doesn't fit into place or feels awkward.

Proper fit also depends on vaginal muscle tone which can change throughout your reproductive years. For this reason, schedule a checkup about once a year or after any of the following events to be sure your diaphragm still fits:

After having a baby (six weeks after delivery).
After a miscarriage or abortion (four weeks afterward).
After pelvic surgery.
Change in weight (loss or gain of 15 pounds or more).
Tension during the initial fitting exam can cause the vaginal muscles to tighten.

After the fitting exam, your doctor or birth control specialist should teach you how to use it. Then you should insert it, remove it, and check its proper position. Be sure to practice this until you can do it correctly, *before* you leave the examining room. While some doctors are reluctant to spend much time teaching women how to use the diaphragm, this is an essential part of the exam. It should receive as much attention—if not more—than the fitting. At the end of the exam, the doctor either writes a prescription for your diaphragm or gives you a diaphragm and spermicide, as part of your office visit fee.

☐ HOW TO USE

Your diaphragm must be in place each time before you have sex. Though you can insert it up to six hours ahead, the closer to intercourse the better. If more than two hours pass before you have sex or if you repeat intercourse, insert another application of spermicide, without removing the diaphragm. If you have an active sex life, you may want to insert your diaphragm before going to bed every night.

The diaphragm is a highly effective method of contraception *only* when used with spermicidal jelly or cream. These chemicals stop and kill sperm. And they provide extra protection at the cervix if your diaphragm gets dislodged during intercourse. Squeeze a two to three inch ribbon (at least one teaspoon) of spermicide on the inside of the cup. Though it makes no difference which side of the dome is against your cervix, most women insert it with the dome side down to keep the spermicide from dropping out. Spread a thin layer onto the side that will be against your cervix and around the rim. More is not necessarily better. In fact, too much may cause the diaphragm to slip around and make it very difficult to insert.

Inserting a diaphragm is almost like inserting a tampon. You can do this in any of several positions: sitting on the edge of a chair or toilet seat; lying flat on your back with knees bent; squatting on the floor; or propping up one leg on a chair or toilet seat. With one hand, pinch the rim of the diaphragm together with your index and middle fingers and thumb. With the other hand, spread the lips of your vagina. Then, insert the diaphragm into your vagina, on an angle toward the back as far as it will go. When it is in place, the back tucks up behind the cervix and the front end fits snugly behind the pubic bone. Check with your finger to be sure the diaphragm covers the cervix. Though insertion

The diaphragm

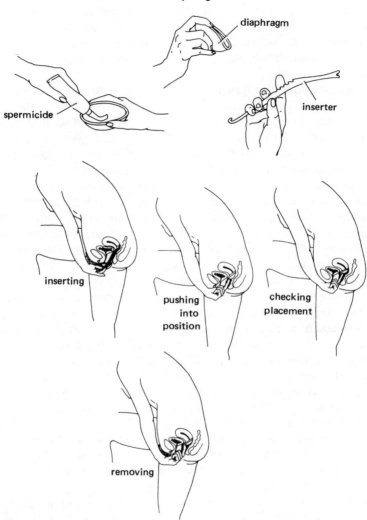

sounds like a lot of trouble, once you learn how to do it, it just takes a few seconds. Also, you are not the only one who can insert it. You and your partner may enjoy including it as part of sexual foreplay.

If you have a retroverted uterus, or dislike handling a messy diaphragm or your genitals, some diaphragms come with a special inserter. The diaphragm, hooked onto the inserter, is pushed in an upward and backward motion along the back of the vagina. To release, give the inserter a quarter turn as you withdraw it.

Remove your diaphragm the following morning or wait at least six hours after your *last* act of intercourse. To remove, hook your finger under the rim and pull downward slowly and gently. Don't douche with the diaphragm in place since it may dilute or flush out the spermicide. If you want to douche, wait until you remove the diaphragm.

When properly cared for, a diaphragm may last two or more years. But it is a good idea to have your diaphragm fit checked every year during your regular pelvic exam. If defects such as puckering, holes, or tears occur, get a new one right away. Once in a while, check your diaphragm for defects by holding it up to the light or by filling it with water to see if drops form on the underside. After removal, wash it in warm water with mild soap, dry it, and dust it with cornstarch. Don't use scented talcs or petroleum jelly since they can weaken a rubber diaphragm. Store it in its compact-like case. If you don't have your container available, temporarily wrap the diaphragm in clean cloth or facial tissue.

Right now there are numerous types of spermicidal jellies and creams available at drugstores without a prescription. Try different brands, since some may cause more discharge than others, or an allergic reaction in either partner, or have an unpleasant smell or taste (for oral-genital sex). If you have tried several brands and your partner still objects to the odor or taste of your spermicide, try washing your vulva with soap and water after inserting the diaphragm.

Both the jellies and creams are water-soluble and nonstaining. Jellies differ from the creams, however. They are colorless, of light consistency, and are more lubricating than cream. (They are good for women with dry vaginal tissues.) Creams are white, of cosmetic-cream consistency, and less lubricating than jelly.

□ SIDE EFFECTS

Even though the diaphragm is nearly 100 percent risk-free, a few men and women develop minor side effects:

> Allergic reaction to rubber.
> Irritation or allergy to spermicide.
> Vaginal infection.

If you or your partner develops an allergic reaction to rubber (local itching or irritation), consult a doctor about a plastic diaphragm. If either one of you develops irritation from a particular spermicide, switch to another brand. Vaginal infection — though rare — may occur if you leave the diaphragm in place more than 24 hours. Call your doctor promptly if you develop this easily-treatable problem.

□ PROS AND CONS

Pros

> Highly effective if properly used.
> Safe, almost 100 percent risk-free.
> Very effective alternative for women who cannot use the Pill or IUD.
> Can be used during menstruation (to control flow during intercourse).
> Can be used during breast-feeding.
> Gives added lubrication during intercourse.
> Good for women who have sex infrequently.

Cons

> Requires a high level of motivation and takes patience and skill to learn how to use.
> Certain women cannot use it.

Requires preparation before intercourse. (Don't run out of spermicide.)

Requires proper fitting by a doctor or birth control specialist.

Is relatively expensive if used frequently due to the cost of the spermicide.

For women uncomfortable about touching their genitals, insertion and removal require genital contact.

Some women view the spermicide as messy (causes slight discharge) and other women view the repeated insertion and removal as a nuisance.

10

CONDOM

For most young couples, the condom — prophylactic, rubber, or safe — is the best starter method of birth control. It also happens to be one of the most effective and widely used barrier methods by American couples of all ages. It literally stops sperm from entering the vagina and uniting with an egg. Speaking of barriers, the condom stops germs as well as sperm: it is prophylactic against sexually-transmitted infections as well as pregnancy. Sexually-transmitted infections can be passed in either direction during sex. The condom protects both the man and the woman against this risk: almost completely against gonorrhea, Trichomonas, Monilia, and Hemophilus vaginitis and offers good protection against syphilis, herpes, and genital warts. The condom has other good things going for it: it can be shared contraception or the closest thing to it. It takes the initiative of the man but allows the participation of the woman during sexual foreplay.

Though the condom is also inexpensive, easy-to-use, and practically 100 percent risk-free, problems exist. The most common complaint is that is interferes with the spontaneity of sex. A lot of men also say it interferes with sexual pleasure by blocking sensation: "It's like taking a shower with a raincoat on." Additionally, it is not a foolproof method. If the condom breaks during intercourse or slips off into the vagina, pregnancy is quite likely. However, if used with a spermicidal foam, it is nearly as effective as the Pill and IUD. To get the most out of this method, your partner has to use a condom *every* time. Equally important is how it is used.

☐ EFFECTIVENESS

Theoretical Effectiveness

Used exactly according to directions, the condom can be 97 percent effective.

Use Effectiveness

Allowing for slip-ups (such as having your partner's condom break during sex), the condom is about 80 percent to 90 percent effective, which is the same as a 10 percent to 20 percent pregnancy rate. This means that if you and your partner use the condom for one year, you have 10 to 20 chances out of one hundred of becoming pregnant.

☐ TYPES

The condom is a very thin but strong, skin-tight sheath worn over an erect penis during intercourse. All U.S.-made ones have to meet quality standards set by the Food and Drug Administration. Basically, there are two types of condoms: rubber and skin. Rubber condoms are the most widely used and least expensive. By comparison, skin condoms (made of lamb's-skin) are not very widely used and cost more than rubber ones. But some men prefer the skin condoms because they seem to interfere less with sensation.

Today's condom buyer has a wide range of styles to choose from. Condoms may be opaque or transparent; tinted just about any color; nipple-ended to catch the semen; rippled; contoured; dry (usually powdered); lubricated; and flocked with a rough rubber surface. The fancy ones cost more but they appeal to many couples. Yet the plain rubber ones are just as good and equally reliable.

Condoms also vary in quality. The best ones are readily

available in drugstores or birth control clinics without a prescription. You can also get condoms through the mail and in vending machines. However, vending machine sales are illegal in half the states. And these condoms are usually of poorer quality and consequently not as reliable as those available in drugstores and clinics.

☐ **HOW TO USE**

Before using a condom, check the date marked on the package and don't use it after that date. If the date is not on the package, use it within two years of the purchase date. A condom usually comes rolled up and sealed in aluminum foil. It should be carefully rolled all the way down the erect penis *before* your partner's penis gets anywhere near your vagina. Believe it or not, one drop of semen can carry sperm and sperm can actually travel from outside the vagina to the uterus and cause pregnancy.

The man doesn't have to be the only one to put the condom on. You and your partner may enjoy including it as part of sexual foreplay. If using a plain-ended condom, leave one-half inch of space at the top without air in it. Then the force of spurting sperm during climax won't tear the condom. If using a reservoir-ended one, the nipple tip catches the semen and helps prevent the condom from bursting. Condoms are also available lubricated or nonlubricated. Some lubrication is necessary to make entry easier and prevent tearing. If your partner uses a nonlubricated condom, apply a lubricant after the condom is on his penis. Use K-Y jelly, saliva, or vaginal spermicide. (Never use petroleum jelly or cold cream since they can weaken the rubber.) If using a lubricated condom, be careful since it can slip off the penis more easily.

After your partner comes to a climax, it is important that he withdraw his penis from your vagina while it is still erect. Your partner should hold the rim of the condom at the base of his penis so it won't slip off and spill semen into your vagina. If the condom tears or slips off into your vagina, use a spermicidal foam. Even though package directions state that you can reuse condoms, it is safer not to. Instead, use a new one every time you have sex.

☐ SIDE EFFECTS

The condom is almost 100 percent risk-free. Yet some men and women develop an allergic reaction (local itching or irritation) to rubber. If this happens, switch to the skin condoms. If either one of you develops irritation from a particular type or style of condom, try different ones.

☐ PROS AND CONS

Pros

Practically 100 percent risk-free.

Readily available in drugstores and birth control clinics without a prescription.

Inexpensive and easy-to-use.

Requires the initiative of the man but allows the participation of the woman during sexual foreplay.

Can be used as a back-up method to provide extra protection during the early months of Pill or IUD use or during midcycle ovulation.

Prophylactic against sexually-transmitted infections. It protects both the man and the woman almost completely against gonorrhea, Trichomonas, Monilia, and Hemophilus vaginitis and provides good protection against syphilis, herpes, and genital warts.

Sometimes sex therapists advise men with premature ejaculation to try the condom since it decreases stimulation of the penis.

Cons

Not always reliable since they can burst under pressure,
leak, or slip off during intercourse.

Air, light, and heat can weaken condoms. They should
not be carried around for months or years in a wal-
let, glove compartment, or stored anywhere it is
warm.

Must be used right at the time of intercourse. For some
couples, this interferes with sexual pleasure and
spontaneity.

The penis must be withdrawn from the vagina right
after ejaculation.

Some men feel that the condom reduces sensitivity and
sensation.

Can be irritating to the woman. (Using lubrication
helps.)

11

VAGINAL SPERMICIDES

Vaginal spermicides come in different forms: foam, jelly, cream, suppositories, or foam tablets. All of these products try to do the same thing. To stop sperm from reaching an egg, a spermicidal substance that destroys sperm covers the opening to the uterus. Some of these products work *much* better than others. In fact, foam is the best. The foam base is really the secret of its success. The pressurized container makes the mixture bubble up. So when foam is inserted into the vagina, it spreads evenly and covers the opening to the uterus. But the other vaginal spermicides have their share of problems. If all goes well, they melt or dissolve to cover the opening to the uterus. Yet, if they don't melt or dissolve (which is often the case) protection is that much less. In fact, when used alone, creams, jellies, suppositories, and foam tablets just don't work. They carry far too great a risk of pregnancy.

☐ EFFECTIVENESS

Of all the vaginal spermicides, *foam* is the most effective. (See Table 10.) *Jelly and cream* should be used only with a diaphragm. Those sold for solo use are less effective than foam. They have a high failure rate, so don't depend on them alone. *Suppositories and foam tablets* are less effective than jelly and cream and much less effective than foam. They have a

TABLE 10. Features of Vaginal Spermicides

Before using any kind of spermicide, read the package brochure *very* carefully. All involve inserting the spermicide high enough into your vagina to cover your cervix. To do this, lie flat on your back with knees bent. With one hand hold the spermicide while your other hand spreads the lips of your vagina. If using an applicator, insert it about three to four inches and push the plunger. If using suppositories or foam tablets, manually place them as high as possible into your vagina.

TYPE	CONSISTENCY	HOW TO USE	WAITING PERIOD FROM INSERTION TO INTERCOURSE*	EFFECTIVENESS†
FOAM	Shaving cream. Distributes evenly.	Shake can 20 times. Fill applicator or use pre-filled applicator.	None	This the *best* spermicide.
JELLY	Clear, light jelly. Melts at body temperature and distributes upon contact with vaginal secretions.	Squeeze tube into applicator	2–3 minutes	Less effective than foam.
CREAM	White, cosmetic cream. Distributes unevenly and remains where it is inserted.	Squeeze tube into applicator or use pre-filled applicator.	2–3 minutes	Less effective than foam and jelly.
SUPPOSITORIES	Gelatin or waxy tablet. If all goes well, they melt at body temperature.	Remove from foil package and insert into vagina or use inserter.	3–15 minutes	*Not very effective at all.*
FOAM TABLETS	White, powdery tablet. If all goes well, they dissolve upon contact with vaginal secretions.	Remove from foil package and insert into vagina. Some require wetting.	3–10 minutes	*Not very effective at all.*

* To increase effectiveness wait for spermicide to melt and distribute in upper vagina and cervix.

† Often, brochures say it is okay to insert spermicide up to an hour before sex. For maximal protection, though, add another application if more than 30 minutes go by without sex or if you stand up to move around or go to the bathroom. Also, add more spermicide each time you have sex again. If you want to douche, wait six to eight hours.

138

very high failure rate, so don't depend on them alone. They are the least effective of all the vaginal spermicides.

Foam is fairly effective when used alone. When used exactly according to directions, foam can be 97 percent effective (theoretical effectiveness). But the trouble is that women sometimes apply foam hurriedly. When used this way, foam is about 75 percent to 85 percent effective (use effectiveness). This means that if you use foam for one year, you have 15 to 25 chances out of one hundred of becoming pregnant. If you use foam with the condom, however, you have a method that is nearly as effective as the IUD.

□ BUYING AND USING

You can buy vaginal spermicides in drugstores without a doctor's prescription. Before buying one, become familiar with the different types and brand names. Often vaginal spermicides are displayed near products that have nothing to do with birth control. To make sure you are buying a contraceptive — and not a feminine hygiene product or vaginal-infection jelly, for example — read the label carefully. Make sure the label says something like "contraceptive foam" on it.

Information contained in patient brochures isn't always helpful either. For example, some companies indicate the product's effectiveness in confusing language: "When pregnancy is medically contraindicated, the contraceptive program should be prescribed by a physician." This means that the product is *not* very effective. Even worse, some companies overpromote their product's effectiveness or only publish theoretical effectiveness data. As a matter of fact, the Food and Drug Administration has received a number of complaints and questions about the effectiveness of Encare Oval — a suppository-like product that came onto the market in late 1977. At first, the promotional literature and consumer labeling described Encare Oval as being 99 percent effective. But after the Food and Drug Administration received serious questions about its effectiveness, the company revised its labeling as of April 1978. Due to unsupported claims about its effectiveness this action became necessary. So be careful when you buy any type of vaginal spermicide. If you have any doubts, consult a pharmacist.

Before using any kind of spermicide, read the directions *very* carefully. Foam, jelly, and cream should be inserted just before intercourse. Suppositories and foam tablets require 5 to 15 minutes before intercourse so they can melt or dissolve. Add more spermicide under these conditions: if more than 30 minutes go by before intercourse; each time you have intercourse again; and if you stand up to move around or go to the bathroom. If you want to douche, wait six to eight hours in order to get the most benefit from your spermicide.

☐ SIDE EFFECTS

Vaginal spermicides are nearly 100 percent risk-free. Occasionally a few men and women develop local irritation or an allergic reaction to one of the spermicides. Usually, the stronger, more effective ones (foam and jelly) tend to be more irritating to the vagina and penis than others. If this happens, try another brand. If the irritation gets severe, see a doctor.

☐ PROS AND CONS

Pros

Inexpensive and easy-to-use.
Safe, almost 100 percent risk-free.
Anyone can buy vaginal spermicides. A doctor's prescription is not necessary.

Vaginal spermicide

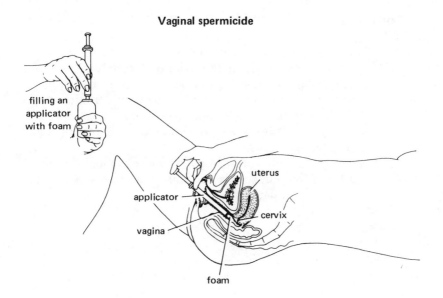

filling an
applicator
with foam

applicator

vagina

uterus

cervix

foam

There is nothing to remove after intercourse.

Menopausal women may find foam provides vaginal lubrication in addition to protecting against late pregnancy.

Interestingly, many foams, jellies, and creams — if inserted before intercourse — provide some protection against gonorrhea and syphilis.

Can be used during breast-feeding.

Pill users planning pregnancy can use foam (and condom) for several months after stopping the Pill until normal menstrual periods resume. (Accidentally taking the Pill during pregnancy may cause birth defects.)

Good for women who have sex infrequently.

Can be used as a back-up method to provide extra protection during the early months of Pill or IUD use or during midcycle ovulation.

Cons

Not highly effective if used alone.

Must be used right at the time of intercourse. All but foam require a waiting period before intercourse.

Must add more spermicide if more than 30 minutes go by before intercourse and each time sex is repeated.

Most spermicides have an unpleasant smell or taste (for oral-genital sex).

Most spermicides are drippy or cause vaginal discharge after intercourse. (Use a tampon after sex if this becomes a problem.)

12

NATURAL BIRTH CONTROL (RHYTHM)

Some women like natural birth control because this method is organic: it doesn't require the use of any drugs or devices, making it 100 percent risk-free. Others subscribe to this method because they are practicing Catholics and natural birth control is still the only acceptable method to the Catholic Church. (A recent study showed that many Catholic women now use other methods.) But natural birth control is not a very reliable method. In fact, every year doctors deliver a lot of unplanned, organic babies due to failures from this method.

In theory, this method is simple: it involves getting to know the rhythm of your menstrual cycles. Basically, you can only become pregnant around the time of ovulation, when the ovary releases an egg. This usually occurs midway between menstrual periods—about 14 days before the start of the next menstrual period. You make this method work by trying to figure out the time of ovulation each month and avoiding sex completely on all the unsafe, fertile days when pregnancy is possible.

Sound too good to be true? Well, it is. This method makes two assumptions, neither of which is true. One, that a woman can tell exactly when ovulation occurs; and two, that sperm have a very short life span. It just so happens that lots of things—such as emotions, physical health, changes in environment, and travel—can affect ovulation. And, even if you were absolutely sure of ovulation, you can't be certain of the life of your partner's sperm. Depending on your vaginal environment, sperm can actually live up to five days waiting for the egg to be released from your ovary.

It is possible to make this method work moderately well, if you really use it carefully. But just looking at the calendar and skipping sex for a few days won't work. This method also won't work if you have irregular menstrual cycles, which 15 percent of all women do. Irregular menstrual cycles are common during puberty and the premenopausal years and for several months after abortion or delivery. (Don't use this method if you fall into any of these categories.)

So, if you want to use natural birth control, see a doctor, birth control clinic, or Planned Parenthood Center first. Only by learning how to use this method correctly and regularly will you get the most protection against pregnancy.

□ TYPES

Right now there are three ways to use natural birth control: with a calendar, a thermometer, or by observing changes in the cervical mucus.

Calendar Method

Of all three methods, this is the oldest one. It also happens to be the least reliable. Though it can be about 85 percent effective when properly used (theoretical effectiveness), most women find it anywhere from 60 percent to 75 percent effective (use effectiveness). This means that if you use the calendar method for one year, you have 25 to 40 chances out of one hundred of becoming pregnant.

By recording the length of your menstrual cycles for eight to twelve months, it is possible to calculate your unsafe, fertile days. You can do this by marking on an ordinary calendar the first day of each menstrual period. (Count the first day of bleeding or spotting as day one of your cycle.)

After you record eight to twelve cycles, calculate the number of days between menstrual periods and use Table 11 as a guide.

For example, if your *shortest* cycle was 26 days and your *longest* cycle was 31 days, then your first unsafe day of every future cycle will be day 8 and your last unsafe day will be day 20. This means that you should avoid intercourse between days 8 to 20 of every month. This is because these are your unsafe, fertile days when pregnancy is possible.

If your longest cycle is ten days longer than your shortest cycle, don't even try to use the calendar method. This method will not work unless your cycles are very regular.

Temperature Method

This method is a lot more reliable than the calendar method. Instead of relying on dates and calendars, the temperature method signals that ovulation has occurred by a small rise in temperature. Properly used, this method can be 90 percent

TABLE 11. How to Calculate the Safe and Unsafe Days

YOUR SHORTEST CYCLE (DAYS)	YOUR FIRST UNSAFE DAY IS	YOUR LONGEST CYCLE (DAYS)	YOUR LAST UNSAFE DAY IS
21	3rd day	21	10th day
22	4th	22	11th
23	5th	23	12th
24	6th	24	13th
25	7th	25	14th
26	8th	26	15th
27	9th	27	16th
28	10th	28	17th
29	11th	29	18th
30	12th	30	19th
31	13th	31	20th
32	14th	32	21st
33	15th	33	22nd
34	16th	34	23rd
35	17th	35	24th

to 95 percent effective (theoretical effectiveness). Allowing for occasional slip-ups, this method has a use effectiveness of about 80 percent, which is the same as a 20 percent pregnancy rate.

By keeping a chart of your body's temperature at rest (basal body temperature), it is possible to detect your time of ovulation. Each morning as soon as you wake up — before getting out of bed, talking, eating, drinking, or smoking — take your temperature. Take your temperature orally or rectally for five full minutes and record your temperature to within 1/10 of a degree on a special basal body temperature chart. (You can get both the thermometer and temperature charts from your local drugstore or birth control clinic.) Generally rectal readings are more reliable than oral ones. Whatever method you choose, take your temperature the same way each day.

As you chart your temperature, you will see how it varies from day to day and even from cycle to cycle. Also realize that illness, tension, or even lack of sleep can affect your basal body temperature, so note down these events on your charts. It will help you interpret your readings. During the early part of the cycle before ovulation, most women have oral temperatures between 96 and 98 degrees. At ovulation, the temperature drops slightly about 0.5 to 1.0 degrees. One to three days later the temperature suddenly rises to a degree *higher than usual* above 98 degrees.

After the temperature rise lasts for at least three days, it is safe to assume that ovulation has taken place. For complete protection, you should only have sex from three days *after* your temperature rise until your next period starts. All of the other days are considered unsafe, fertile days when pregnancy is possible.

Cervical Mucus Method

Also called the Ovulation or Billings method, this is the newest method of natural birth control. It is a system that has to do with recognizing changes in the mucus secretions

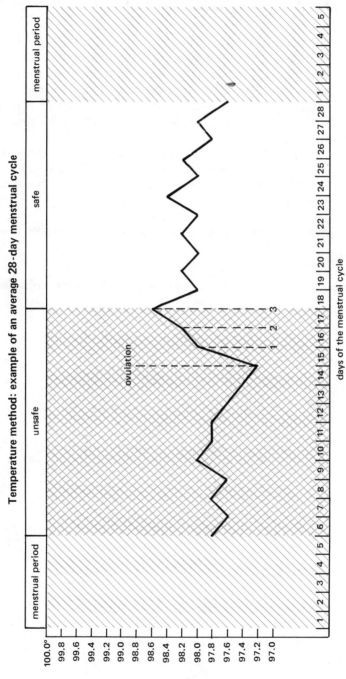

Temperature method: example of an average 28-day menstrual cycle

from the cervix. Though this recent method has received lots of publicity, it's so new that it is still under study. In fact, it is really too early to make statements about the reliability of the cervical mucus method. The few studies to date report that it is anywhere from 75 percent to 97 percent effective, which is the same as a 3 percent to 25 percent pregnancy rate.

With proper instructions, women can learn to associate changes in the volume and consistency of their cervical mucus at different points in their menstrual cycle. Basically, this system goes like this:

The cycle begins with menstruation. The days while

Cervical mucus method: example of an average 28-day menstrual cycle

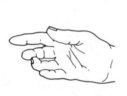

Dry, no mucus.
Infertile, safe days.

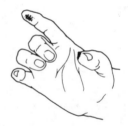

Cloudy, thick, sticky.
Beginning of unsafe days.

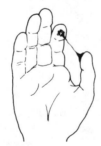

Ovulation:
Profuse, clear, stringy.
Fertile, unsafe days.

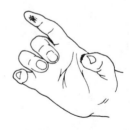

Cloudy, thick, tacky.
Infertile, safe days.

bleeding lasts are considered *unsafe*. Should ovulation occur, menstrual bleeding would hide the mucus signs.

After the menstrual period, there may be a few "dry" days when there is no mucus. If these days occur, they are considered *safe*.

As an egg starts to ripen, mucus appears that is sticky, and cloudy white or yellow. This is the beginning of the "wet," *unsafe* days, when you should avoid sex.

Just before ovulation, the mucus increases in amount, and becomes clear and slippery, like raw eggs. You can stretch it between your fingers. These "wet" days are the *peak of fertility* when you should avoid sex.

The longest *safe* period begins on the fourth day after the mucus peak and lasts until the next menstrual period.

Many — but not all — women experience all of these changes. In fact, about 30 percent of all women don't have clear-cut changes. If you are interested in trying this new method, get instructions from a birth control clinic familiar with this technique. You will be taught how to sample and make daily recordings of your cervical mucus. You can do this by inserting a finger into your vagina; touching your cervix with your fingertips; observing discharge on your underpants; or by wiping your vagina with tissue.

This method becomes less reliable if you douche, use vaginal spermicides, have a vaginal infection, are approaching your menopause, or had surgery on your cervix. As with all the other methods of natural birth control, this one requires careful record-keeping.

Combined Methods

To increase effectiveness and to increase the number of days it is safe to have sex, some couples combine methods. For example, couples who object to using birth control devices at any time combine two methods of natural birth control.

Other couples use natural birth control plus an effective mechanical method (such as foam and condom) on the unsafe, fertile days.

Temperature and Calendar Methods. One possibility is to combine the temperature and calendar methods. For the temperature method, you keep your temperature graph in the regular way. For the calendar method, you also need to mark every day one on a calendar and keep a record of the number of days in each cycle. Let's say your shortest cycle is 26 days. This means that your first unsafe day is day nine. (See Table 11.) From then on, don't have sex until after the third day of your temperature rise. While many couples find this an acceptable method, it is not as effective as the temperature method alone.

Temperature and Cervical Mucus Methods. Another possibility is to combine the temperature and cervical mucus methods. Changes in cervical mucus are usually obvious before a temperature rise, so the signs of one serve to confirm the signals of the other. The same rules apply here for temperature taking and noting cervical mucus changes. Having a record of mucus changes can be quite helpful when temperatures rise from illness, emotional upset, or lack of sleep. This method has an added bonus: it shortens the period of abstinence necessary for complete protection when using the temperature method alone. Also called the "Sympto-Thermal" method, preliminary studies show that this method can be about 93 percent effective.

☐ PROS AND CONS

Pros

> Safe, 100 percent risk-free.
> After initial costs, there are no other expenses.
> Requires no preparation at the time of intercourse.

Promotes understanding of reproduction and the menstrual cycle.

An alternative for couples who cannot — for religious, medical, or personal reasons — use birth control devices or drugs.

Can lead to exploring other intimate forms of sexual pleasure during the unsafe days.

Couples *desiring* pregnancy often use the temperature method to find the most fertile days when sex will most likely result in pregnancy.

Cons

Least effective method of birth control.

Women with irregular cycles cannot use this method.

Can create anxiety about pregnancy and interfere with sexual spontaneity.

Expert medical guidance is necessary to make this method work.

Requires a high level of patience and motivation by both partners.

Depending on the method, must avoid sex from one to three weeks of every cycle. Many couples find this sexually frustrating.

Requires careful daily record-keeping.

Is a method that requires calendars, charts, graphs, and thermometers really natural?

13

OTHER METHODS AND NONMETHODS

☐ **OTHER METHODS**

Withdrawal

Being careful or getting out in time means withdrawing the penis from the vagina just before ejaculation. Luck and perfect timing are essential so that your partner does not deposit any sperm into your vagina, or anywhere near it. Believe it or not, sperm can travel up into the vagina from its outer edge.

Though some people say that withdrawal is as effective as the diaphragm and the condom, you need considerable motivation and self-control to reach that kind of effectiveness. Even if you exercise great care, there is a risk factor with this method 25 percent of the time. Right after your partner's penis becomes erect, sperm can escape — without your partner's knowledge — into your vagina before he comes to a climax, causing pregnancy. Also, if you repeat intercourse shortly after, pregnancy is possible since surviving sperm from the surface of the penis are mixed with the lubricating fluid.

Additionally, many couples find withdrawal emotionally unsatisfying. Not only is it difficult to relax but it interrupts the excitement phase of intercourse, which can greatly reduce pleasure for both the man and the woman. On the plus

153

side, this method is free and without any health risks. It is also a method that is always available. Even so, be skeptical of male confidence, unless you know your partner well. Better yet, choose a less frustrating and more reliable method of birth control.

Morning-After Contraception

Maybe you have heard there is something you can do to actually prevent pregnancy if you have intercourse at midcycle without contraception. It's true. There is the morning-after pill and the morning-after IUD. Used no later than three days after unprotected intercourse, these methods seem to work well. But they are not *routine* methods for regular or repeated use. In fact, they are methods only worth considering in case of an emergency.

Morning-After Pill. In February 1975 the Food and Drug Administration (FDA) approved *limited* use of stilbestrol, known as DES, as a contraceptive agent for midcycle sexual exposure. (Even so, the FDA has not yet approved a marketing application for postcoital use of DES. See Chapter 16, The Stilbestrol Problem.) According to the FDA, DES should be used "for emergencies only and should not be used routinely." While some college-age women tend to overuse the morning-after pill, it should be used only for cases of rape, incest, or similar medical emergencies.

But DES is not a new drug. Doctors have used it since the 1940s to treat a number of medical conditions. Until 1971 it was widely used to prevent miscarriage and to treat the high-risk pregnancy. But in that year, researchers associated DES during pregnancy with cancer of the vagina and cervix in DES-exposed daughters. Since then, the FDA has prohibited the use of DES for treatment of the high-risk pregnancy.

Right now there is no evidence that DES taken one to three days after intercourse will cause cancer in exposed daughters if the morning-after pill fails. There is, however, ample evidence that female fetuses exposed to DES during the sixth week of pregnancy or later are at higher risk for developing cancer during adolescence or later. Time of DES exposure is crucial to the possible development of genital conditions. Between the sixth and twelfth week of pregnancy, the genital tract is forming in the embryo and it is extremely sensitive to agents which could cause birth defects. Yet, if DES is taken one to three days after intercourse, a fluid-filled ball of cells—rather than the genital tract—is exposed to DES.

If you qualify as an emergency and want to take the morning-after pill, go to your doctor or clinic preferably within 24 hours, but no later than 72 hours after unprotected intercourse. If you go later than this, DES will not prevent pregnancy. This is because the morning-after pill works by preventing implantation of an egg after fertilization has taken place. (A fertilized egg usually reaches the uterus in four to five days.) Before giving you a prescription for the morning-after pill, the doctor should take your medical history and perform a gynecologic physical exam. If you can take DES, the doctor will prescribe 25 mg pills of DES to be taken twice a day for five days. This extremely high dose of estrogen often causes nausea as well as vomiting. Other side effects may include breast tenderness, headaches, and menstrual irregularities.

Though the morning-after pill seems to work well, it won't work if you are already pregnant; if you don't take all the pills or vomit some of them; or have unprotected intercourse after taking all your pills. If your menstrual period is two weeks late after taking your pills, arrange a pregnancy test. If DES fails, the FDA advises you to consider having an abortion due to the potential cancer risk to DES-exposed female fetuses.

Morning-After IUD. If you cannot or don't want to take DES, having a copper IUD inserted after unprotected intercourse will also prevent pregnancy. This is the latest method of morning-after contraception. In fact, it is so new that it is currently under study and not yet approved by the FDA. In one study, nearly 100 women had a Copper-7 inserted after unprotected intercourse. No pregnancies occurred. As a result of these promising findings, more and more gynecologists now use copper IUDs for this purpose.

If you want to use this method, go to a doctor or clinic that inserts morning-after IUDs, no later than three days after unprotected intercourse. Like the morning-after pill, the IUD works by preventing implantation of an egg after fertilization has taken place. If your menstrual period is two weeks late after having an IUD inserted, arrange a pregnancy test.

The advantage of the IUD over the morning-after pill is that it doesn't cause nausea, vomiting, or the potentially dangerous side effects found with DES. Another obvious advantage is that — once the IUD is inserted — it can be used in the future as a method of contraception. But the morning-after IUD is not totally without risk. The usual contraindications to IUD insertion apply here. (See Table 7.) Women who are pregnant or have pelvic inflammatory disease or gonorrhea should definitely *not* use the morning-after IUD since it could result in serious complications.

Abstinence

There is always abstinence or just not having intercourse at all. In fact, there are times when it becomes desirable or necessary to leave sex out altogether. Or you can substitute intercourse for exploring other intimate forms of sexual pleasure such as mutual masturbation or oral-genital sex. It has the obvious advantage of being an extremely effective, 100 percent risk-free method of birth control. It is not — as some people say — bad for you. It can be a healthy, respectable option, especially for short periods of time. But abstinence is only good when you freely choose it. Not choosing it can be a depriving, lonely experience.

☐ NONMETHODS

Douching

Douching or washing out the vagina after intercourse is a worthless, folk-method of birth control. You may get a nice clean feeling afterward, but hardly any protection against pregnancy. Yet over the years, solutions such as water, soap suds, vinegar, lemon juice, and Coca Cola have been popular as post-intercourse douches. Besides being ineffective, douching may even irritate the vaginal tissues.

Trying to remove sperm from the vagina before they reach the uterus is an impossible task. Sperm swim faster than you can reach the bathroom. In addition, squirting liquid into the vagina actually encourages some sperm to swim into the uterus, even though others are washed out.

All in all, don't use douching to prevent pregnancy. It just doesn't work.

Breast-Feeding

Worldwide, many women rely on breast-feeding as a method of birth control after delivery. This is because breast-feeding protects against pregnancy by delaying the return of ovulation and menstrual periods. It seems that women who breast-feed full-time *may* not ovulate for about eight to twelve months after delivery. (Women who don't breast-feed ovulate about two to four months after delivery.) And when you don't ovulate, pregnancy is impossible.

While breast-feeding tends to work — at least in some women — it is impossible to predict when ovulation will return. Your *first* menstrual period after delivery signals that ovulation has returned. Yet many women ovulate before their first menstrual period, making breast-feeding a very unreliable method of birth control.

If you choose to breast-feed after delivery, be sure to discuss contraception with your doctor. If you used a diaphragm before pregnancy, it won't fit. (You have to wait six weeks after delivery before getting a new one.) In the meantime, you can use foam and condom or consider having an IUD inserted. (Often IUDs are inserted right after delivery or eight weeks later.) If you want to use the birth control pill during breast-feeding, consider the minipill. Unlike estrogen containing pills, minipills do not reduce the amount of breast milk.

Other

You may have heard that you can't get pregnant when you:

> Avoid having an orgasm.
> Don't have sex lying down.
> Have sex during your menstrual period.
> Have sex when your periods are not regular during adolescence and the menopausal years.

Forget what you have heard. These are worthless ineffective methods of birth control. You can become pregnant if you rely on any one of them. Choose a real method of birth control — one that works.

14

STERILIZATION

If you are looking for a virtually foolproof and permanent method of birth control, voluntary sterilization may be the answer. But sterilization is not for everyone. For this reason, you and your partner should carefully discuss your decision with your doctor or birth control specialist. Then you must both decide which of you is to have the operation. Generally, the man or woman most strongly in favor of permanent fertility termination is the best candidate for voluntary sterilization.

It is essential that you or your partner *freely choose* to undergo sterilization: without any outside pressure, either for or against the operation. Moreover, you should also know that:

> According to recent statistics, over nine million American men and women have already chosen sterilization for contraceptive reasons. More couples than ever before now choose sterilization for any of the following reasons: if no pregnancies are desired in the future; if pregnancy is likely to endanger a woman's physical or emotional health; if there is a possibility of transmitting a hereditary defect; reluctance to use temporary birth control for 20 years or more; and concern over the possible long-term effects of using the Pill or IUD.
>
> Sterilization is now legal in all states. While there are no state or federal laws requiring consent of a spouse,

many doctors and hospitals do request the spouse's consent.

As a patient, you have the right to complete information so that you can give your "informed consent" before undergoing sterilization. Informed consent should entail an explanation of the sterilization procedure, its risks, benefits, and alternative types of procedures that exist for you. Informed consent may be verbal but is usually written. Both forms are legally valid.

Sterilization is generally irreversible and permanent. Though researchers are currently improving techniques for surgical restoration of fertility, doctors cannot guarantee successful reversal for anyone. For this reason, don't choose sterilization if you hope to have your fertility restored in case of remarriage, divorce, or death of children.

Sterilization does not affect a person's sexual enjoyment or sex organs. Other than the inability to reproduce, there are no known physical changes in women. A woman's menstrual periods, hormone levels, and age of menopause remain unaffected, unless hysterectomy is done. Likewise, a man continues to produce male hormones and have erections, orgasms, and ejaculations of semen as much as before, but the semen is sperm-free.

Sterilization will not solve emotional, sexual, or relationship problems. In fact, men and women who view sterilization as a problem-solver frequently develop personal problems after surgery.

After all is said and done—if your decision is sterilization— be sure to have your surgery done by a doctor experienced in sterilization procedures. If your doctor is not experienced in this area, ask for a referral to a doctor who is. Or, if you prefer, you can contact your local Planned Parenthood Center or the Association for Voluntary Sterilization for assistance. (See Readings and Resources.)

☐ METHODS FOR WOMEN

Tubal Sterilization

Right now there are several methods of tubal sterilization. Regardless of the method used, the result is always the same: the Fallopian tubes are closed off to prevent the passage of eggs from the ovaries to the uterus. Sometimes the tubes are closed off by cutting and/or tying (tubal ligation); burning and sealing (cautery); or applying clips or bands. When this happens, your eggs cannot meet your partner's sperm, making fertilization of a sperm and an egg next to impossible.

Laparotomy. Until recently sterilization required major surgery, several days stay in the hospital, and nearly several weeks of recuperation at home. This is because laparotomy — a three to four inch incision in the abdomen — was necessary to locate and cut and/or tie the tubes. Though laparotomy is still practiced, most doctors have turned their attention to simpler methods of sterilization.

While laparotomy may be done at any time, doctors commonly perform it right after delivery or other surgery such as cesarean section or abortion. Done at this time, a separate hospital admission becomes unnecessary.

Common side effects following laparotomy — which are not serious and disappear in several days with treatment — may include tenderness or infection at the incision.

Mini-Laparotomy. Unlike laparotomy, this new technique requires only a one-inch incision in the abdomen to locate the Fallopian tubes. Through the incision the tubes are either cut and/or tied or closed with clips or bands. This simplified procedure substantially reduces recovery time, thus making it possible to offer the "mini-lap" on an outpatient basis with local anesthesia. If you have any of the following medical conditions, you should not undergo mini-laparotomy: extreme overweight; pelvic infection; history of extensive pelvic surgery; or endometriosis.

With the exception of tenderness at the incision, mini-laparotomy is generally without side effects.

Laparoscopy. Many medical centers and clinics are now pioneering a new, much simpler method of sterilization. Often called "Band-Aid" or "belly-button" surgery, laparoscopy is now the most popular method of sterilization for women. It is a technique that allows a well-trained doctor to view the abdomen with a laparoscope, a pencil-like viewing device with a light source.

To see the organs clearly, the abdomen is inflated with a harmless gas (carbon dioxide). Through one or two small incisions in the abdomen the doctor inserts the laparoscope and an instrument to close off the Fallopian tubes. Usually the tubes are sealed with a cauterizing instrument. But some doctors are now applying new, specially-designed clips or bands to the tubes. Made of either plastic or metal, the spring-loaded clips grip the tubes tightly shut, while the silicone bands squeeze the tubes shut like an ordinary rubber band. More and more doctors now use both devices since they make sterilization safer by eliminating the risk of injury to nearby organs with a cauterizing instrument. Moreover, if you want corrective tubal surgery at a later date, clips and bands have a higher reversibility rate than cauterization.

An increasing number of medical centers and clinics now offer laparoscopy on an out-patient basis with local anesthesia. Laparoscopy is also commonly performed right after abortion or delivery. However, if you have any of the following medical conditions, you should not undergo laparoscopy: extreme overweight; hernia; history of extensive pelvic surgery; heart disease; or respiratory disease.

Side effects of laparoscopy may include discomfort and shoulder pain from the carbon dioxide introduced into the abdomen and tenderness from the incision. Cauterization can also cause a brief, sharp pain as it seals the Fallopian tubes.

Culdoscopy and Colpotomy. In less commonly performed methods, sterilization is done through the vagina instead of the abdomen. Culdoscopy — similar to laparoscopy — is a technique that allows a well-trained doctor to view the abdomen with a culdoscope, a pencil-like viewing instrument with a light on the end. Through a small incision in the vagina, the doctor inserts the culdoscope to close off the Fallopian tubes. Usually the tubes are cut and/or tied, but sometimes doctors apply clips to them. Colpotomy is similar to culdoscopy except that a viewing instrument is not used.

As cosmetically appealing as these methods may sound, they are not problem-free. Not only are they more difficult to perform than other methods, they are also not without medical risks. For this reason they are never done right after abortion or delivery. Moreover, women with any of the following medical conditions should not undergo culdoscopy: infection of the vagina or cervix; pelvic inflammatory disease; extreme overweight; growths such as endometriosis or fibroids; heart disease; or respiratory disease. Contraindications to colpotomy include: pelvic infection; extreme overweight; abdominal growths or adhesions; and women who have never delivered a baby.

Hysterectomy

Until recently, hysterectomy — surgical removal of the uterus — was the most common method of sterilization. According to estimates, sterilization is still one of the major reasons for hysterectomy in women under age 40. Yet hysterectomy for contraception alone represents unnecessary surgery. This is just one of the features that makes hysterectomy the target of public criticism and the focus of medical controversy. Most importantly, hysterectomy is currently one of the most overused and costly surgical procedures, not without medical risks.

Hysterectomy is *not* a routine procedure for sterilization. It should only be reserved for women *desiring* sterilization who *also* have an existing gynecologic problem such as endometriosis or fibroids that causes pain and bleeding. See Chapter 18 for other gynecologic conditions that may require hysterectomy. Most importantly, if a doctor recommends hysterectomy as a method of sterilization, get a second surgical opinion about the necessity of hysterectomy.

☐ METHODS FOR MEN

Vasectomy

More and more men are taking advantage of vasectomy, a minor surgical procedure that now ranks as one of the simplest and most popular methods of sterilization. To reach the sperm-carrying tubes (vas deferens), the doctor makes one or two small incisions in the sack containing the testicles (scrotum). Usually the tubes are cut and tied. But some doctors now block the tubes with cautery or specially-designed clips.

This 10 to 20 minute procedure can be done at any time in the doctor's office, clinic, or hospital under local anesthesia. With the exception of local pain and swelling for a day or two, vasectomy is usually without complications.

For some time after vasectomy, the fluid ejaculated at sexual climax (semen) is not sperm-free. This is because sperm remain in the vas deferens before vasectomy and therefore come out in the semen after the operation. For this reason, you and your partner need to use another method of birth control until the semen becomes sperm-free. This varies from man to man. Generally there are no sperm in the semen 15 ejaculations after vasectomy. If laboratory analysis of the semen still shows sperm, repeat semen specimens are necessary until two consecutive sperm counts are sperm-free.

☐ REVERSING STERILIZATION

Until recently the results of sterilization operations were considered permanent and irreversible. But a growing number of people who remarry or simply change their minds are now having their procedures reversed. By means of microsurgical techniques, surgeons at a few U.S. medical centers are able to satisfy their demands: at least some of the time. Fertility experts estimate that several thousand men and women seek sterilization reversals every year. These experts warn, however, that good results can *never* be guaranteed.

While sterilization for men and women can usually be done in a doctor's office or clinic under local anesthesia, surgery to restore fertility takes several hours under general anesthesia. Moreover, it is far more expensive than a sterilization procedure and can require up to a week's stay in the hospital. Before attempting this operation on a woman, most surgeons examine the Fallopian tubes with a laparoscope to see if reversal is possible. If it is, the surgeon goes ahead with the operation. With the help of a surgical microscope, the doctor opens the cut ends of the tubes and stitches them back together with sutures. Women who were sterilized by tubal ligation, where the tubes are cut and/or tied, have about a 60 percent chance of being made fertile again with this operation. (The reversibility rate with clips and bands is also fairly high, yet it is still too early to determine how high.) But the operation isn't nearly as successful for women who have undergone the increasingly popular "Band-Aid" surgery (laparoscopy), where the tubes are burned and sealed with a cauterizing instrument. It turns out that less than 10 percent of all women sterilized with cautery can have their fertility restored. Male vasectomy reversal is no more difficult than reversing tubal ligation in women. Here, the fertility success rate is about 45 percent — and sometimes higher — when fertility is restored with microsurgery.

Regardless of how encouraging these statistics may sound, be sure to weigh your decision to undergo sterilization very seriously. Though researchers are currently working on techniques for surgical restoration of fertility, doctors *cannot* guarantee successful reversal for anyone. For this reason, you should view sterilization as irreversible and permanent. Never undergo it if you hope to have your fertility restored in the future.

15

ABORTION

Until recently abortion was illegal for most women. Though one-third of the U.S. states liberalized their abortion laws from 1967 to 1970, it wasn't until the Supreme Court's 1973 decision that all U.S. women were given the legal right to get an abortion "on request"; that is, for any reason.

The 1973 abortion laws as they now stand say that you are entitled to an abortion by a licensed doctor through your second trimester of pregnancy. Specifically, this means that:

> Through the first trimester of pregnancy, abortion is a decision made *solely* between you and your doctor.
>
> During the second trimester, "the State, in promoting its interest" in the woman's health, may only impose regulations that are "reasonably related to maternal health;" that is, regulations that will safeguard your health.
>
> After the second trimester, the State may regulate or even prohibit abortion except when it is necessary to preserve your life or health.

Prior to these laws, women with money could get an abortion: in foreign countries where abortions were obtained easily; by paying a high price to a private doctor; or by being admitted to a hospital for a D and C for "female troubles." Women without money went to back-alley abortionists or midwives who performed nonmedical abortions under unsanitary conditions, not to mention the high rate of complications, infection, infertility, and even death.

Many organizations influenced the abortion reform movement in the 1960s: National Abortion Rights Action League, Planned Parenthood, Clergy Consultation Service, American Civil Liberties Union, the women's movement, and so forth. These groups, committed to the issue of abortion, joined the fight for reform by carrying out activities in research, education, and public service. Other groups issued position statements.

Alongside these groups and organizations, other groups opposed the Supreme Court's decision. They opposed it so much that they are still pushing for constitutional amendments to overturn the current abortion laws. These "right to life" groups argue that a fetus is a person from the moment of conception and, for this reason, has a right to be protected from "murder." The Catholic Church — often associated with an anti-abortion position — is a major financial contributor to the right to life movement. Anti-abortion organizations at the national level, to name just a few, include: Birthright, Lifeline, and National Right to Life. Such diverse groups as the Salvation Army, the Church of Jesus Christ of Latter-Day Saints (Mormons), Protestant fundamentalists, and Black Muslims, are also among the anti-abortion forces. These groups, which have conducted an energetic public relations campaign, are currently trying to receive more favorable publicity from the media than the pro-abortion movement.

If you are pregnant with an unplanned pregnancy, there are alternatives available to you. Legal abortion is now one of these alternatives, wherever you live in the United States. If your decision is abortion, this chapter guides you through the process. If, however, you prefer to continue your pregnancy, realize that women of all ages, races, backgrounds, religions, interests, and marital status do just that. As reactions to unplanned pregnancies vary, so do the choices and decisions. Some women want an abortion and that is all there is to it. To others, the thought alone may be wrong.

Think about what you want to do; what suits you best. Also realize — as a result of the Supreme Court's decision — you now have the right to choose: "Should I continue with my pregnancy?" or "Should I get an abortion?" You now have the basic right to choose whether and when to have your children.

☐ DIAGNOSIS OF PREGNANCY

Your menstrual period is late: not a day or two, but a week or so. Maybe you have had late or missed periods during times of stress, illness, or fatigue. But this time you feel different. Your breasts may be tender and enlarged; you may feel exhausted and need more sleep than usual; or have nausea and/or vomiting, especially in the morning. If you have some of these symptoms, and had sexual intercourse last month, you may be pregnant. If you think you are pregnant, wait 10 to 14 days from the day your period was due, because with currently available tests it takes that long for pregnancy to be detected. Then arrange to get a medical pregnancy diagnosis: not just a test done on your urine but an internal examination of your uterus by your doctor or clinic.

First, you need to get a laboratory test done on your urine that checks for a hormone (chorionic gonadotrophin) made by the body during early pregnancy. This test is effective about two weeks after your missed period. Two new blood tests — radioimmunoassay and radioreceptorassay — have made pregnancy detection possible even before a missed period. Unfortunately, they are too expensive for general use in doctor's offices and clinics and — for this reason — are only available in well-equipped hospitals and medical centers. Secondly, you need to arrange an appointment with your doctor or clinic for an internal exam of your uterus to confirm the diagnosis of pregnancy.

Maybe you know a doctor with whom you can discuss your possible pregnancy. If so, you can have your urine test and pelvic exam done all at once. If you do not have your own doctor or if you are uneasy about calling your doctor, there are alternatives available to you. For pregnancy testing, you can call any of the following agencies for information or testing.

Planned Parenthood. Many Planned Parenthood Centers provide pregnancy testing, in addition to other birth control services. (See Readings and Resources.) Consult the White Pages for the Planned Parenthood Center in your community.

Local Hospital Gynecology Clinic. Many hospitals have free or low-cost gynecology clinics where you can arrange a pregnancy test. Call your local hospital and ask to speak with the nurse in charge of the gynecology clinic.

Local Health Department. Call your local health department listed in the phone book. If they can't provide a urine test, they can refer you to a hospital that will do it.

Family Planning Center or Women's Health Clinic. Call your local family planning center or women's health clinic listed in the Yellow Pages under: Clinics; Family Planning Information Centers; or Pregnancy Information Service. If they can't provide a urine test, they will refer you to a place that can do it.

Medical Laboratory. Consult the Yellow Pages for: Laboratory, Medical; or Pregnancy Tests. Laboratories vary greatly in quality. Be sure to use a certified laboratory. If you are doubtful, consult your local family planning center or women's health clinic for the lab's reputation. Also, some labs will not give the results directly to you, but only to your doctor, hospital, or clinic.

Do-It-Yourself Pregnancy Test. It is now possible to buy one of several do-it-yourself tests at your local drugstore, without a prescription. These kits have attractive features. You test your urine privately at home without waiting for a medical appointment. In addition, you can start testing yourself for pregnancy on the ninth day after your missed period, instead of the conventional two weeks with most medical laboratory tests. Do-it-yourself tests have a bad history, though. In 1972, the Food and Drug Administration prohibited the sale of a test called Ova II. This action became necessary when the test was found to be "inaccurate, unreliable, and prone to give false results." It turns out that Ova II was about 50 percent accurate. It missed a correct diagnosis of pregnancy 50 percent of the time. On the contrary, standard medical laboratory tests are 97 percent to 99 percent accurate.

Since early 1978 it has been possible to buy a test called e.p.t. (early pregnancy test). This test has been around the longest, but there are also a few others. Though e.p.t. is similar to most tests done in medical laboratories, it is not without problems. While the e.p.t. advertisements claim accuracy as early as the ninth day after the missed menstrual period, it is only accurate for positive tests. When it is positive, it is 97 percent accurate for pregnancy. Yet when it is negative, it is only 80 percent accurate. This means that e.p.t. misses a diagnosis of pregnancy in 20 percent of all women. That many "false-positives" do not make e.p.t. very reliable. Moreover, e.p.t., which is not reusable, is more expensive than a medical laboratory test. Even if the test result is accurate, you still have to see a doctor for an internal examination of your uterus (and most likely another pregnancy test) to confirm the diagnosis of pregnancy.

While all women have the basic right to information about their own fertility as simply and privately as possible, be sure to consider the pros and cons of do-it-yourself tests before deciding to use one.

University Health Service. Some colleges and universities provide birth control, pregnancy testing, and abortion referral services as part of their health program. If you feel this impinges on your privacy, use another facility.

Instructions for collecting your urine sample vary from place to place. If you choose to have your urine test and pelvic exam done all at once, the doctor or clinic will ask for a urine sample when you arrive or ask you to bring a container of your first morning urine. If you choose to have the urine test done as a separate procedure at a certified medical laboratory, you should deliver a container of your first morning urine. Many medications and drugs can cause a urine test to appear positive when it may be negative. For this reason, if you are currently taking any medications or drugs, mention it to the person giving you the test.

A urine test can be positive, negative, or doubtful. If it is positive, you can assume you are pregnant. You should arrange to see a doctor or clinic to confirm pregnancy with a pelvic exam. If both these tests confirm pregnancy, your doctor will determine how many weeks pregnant you are. This is calculated by counting the number of weeks from the first day of your last menstrual period (LMP) and not the day you actually became pregnant. For example, if your period is two weeks late and your menstrual cycle is about 28 days long, you are considered six weeks pregnant, even though you are really only four weeks pregnant.

If the test is negative or doubtful, you are probably not pregnant, but "false-negatives" can happen, especially with do-it-yourself tests. If you have a negative or doubtful result —from *any* type of pregnancy test—and your menstrual period does not arrive in another week, consult your doctor or clinic about a second pregnancy test.

□ DECISION-MAKING

You are pregnant. Also surprised, since you didn't plan it. Now you have to deal with your feelings about being pregnant: "Should I get an abortion?" or "Should I continue with my pregnancy?" You know that having a baby at this time would be a disaster for you and for others. Feeling trapped, frightened, and desperate, you know that an abortion is the right thing for you — or is it? You are doubtful, angry, guilty, and at times very sad.

You continue to move back and forth from one decision to the next and back again — truly having difficulty with your mixed feelings. You are also afraid of any kind of surgery, especially abortion with its long back-alley history when abortions were illegal, even though they are now legal and safe. Your thoughts continue: will it hurt, will I get some awful complication, will I become sterile, or will I later have regrets and wish I had the baby, where will I get the money, or there goes my career.

All of these fears are normal. Many women have felt some, maybe all of them. But fear can arise from lack of knowledge about what really takes place, or from bits of information, or from totally false information. Once you learn what takes place, you will be less afraid, less anxious, and better able to cope.

You need to talk to someone: someone you can trust, someone who will listen, and someone who will not try to persuade you one way or another. For some women, this may be a doctor, a nurse, or a female friend. For others, it may be a favorite school teacher, professor, or guidance counselor. Maybe you can talk to your partner or parents. Though you should try to share your feelings with your partner, try to realize that the people you are closest to and who love you the most, often lose sight of how to help you at this time.

Maybe you don't know anyone who can help you get a clear view of what is involved in abortion, help you examine your feelings, and help you come to your own decision. If this is your situation, consider getting in touch with Planned Parenthood or another nonprofit agency for counseling and advice.

If your decision is abortion, an abortion referral agency can tell you where to go and what to do. (More about that later.) If you choose to continue your pregnancy, you have three alternatives: keep your baby; give your baby to another family temporarily (foster home); or give up your baby permanently (adoption). You can call your own doctor, clinic, or Planned Parenthood to find out where to get prenatal care, financial support, or help in arranging an adoption or foster home.

Whatever your state of mind, don't wait. If you decide to have an abortion, the earlier you decide the easier it will be physically, emotionally, and financially.

☐ ABORTION REFERRAL AGENCIES

Despite the 1973 Supreme Court decision legalizing doctor-performed abortions through the second trimester of pregnancy in all 50 states, getting an abortion is not a simple matter in certain parts of the country. This is because there are still not enough places performing abortions at reasonable costs. Moreover, the people opposed to abortion have adopted restrictive guidelines or — even worse — have refused to perform abortions at all.

Where your abortion takes place depends on a number of factors: how many weeks pregnant you are; where you live; your age; your abortion referral source; how much you can afford; and what your health insurance will cover.

Information about where and how to get an abortion can be obtained from many good — and some not so good — abortion referral agencies. Advertisements for agencies can be found in many college, underground, city, and small town newspapers and magazines. Many of these showy ads represent commercial, profit-making abortion referral agencies that charge you for their service and/or get kickbacks from the doctors or clinics they use for referrals. Some, but not all, have been prosecuted and closed down. Unless you are reliably referred to a commercial agency, choose carefully. Better yet, get in touch with any of the following noncommercial, nonprofit abortion referral services that provide free consultation and referral.

Planned Parenthood

Planned Parenthood offers a variety of services — abortion, pregnancy testing, venereal disease, contraception, sterilization, infertility, and related services — in almost every state. (See Readings and Resources.) In addition to contraception, which all of them provide, many Planned Parenthood Centers offer pregnancy testing, and some perform abortions. If the Planned Parenthood in your area does not perform abortions, they can refer you to a clinic, hospital, or doctor's office that does. Planned Parenthood keeps excellent follow-up records on hundreds of competent doctors, clinics, and hospitals performing abortions in well-equipped and well-staffed facilities nationwide.

Information (medical and legal) and abortion referral are free. There may be a charge for counseling. Consult the phone book for the Planned Parenthood Center in your community. If you can't find a listing, call information in your state capital since many Planned Parenthood Centers are located in state capitals and other metropolitan areas. Or call their central office in New York City.

Family Planning Center or Women's Health Clinic

Numerous nonprofit agencies provide free abortion information and referral. Consult the Yellow Pages for: Clinics; Family Planning Information Centers; or Pregnancy Information Services.

Other

Some colleges and universities provide abortion information and referral as part of their health program. If you feel this impinges on your privacy, use another service. Or, if you have been reliably referred to a private doctor, you may wish to consult that doctor for your abortion or a referral.

Moreover, you should know that Clergy Consultation Service and Zero Population Growth — once active nonprofit abortion referral services at the national level — no longer provide this service. Clergy Consultation Service was formed in 1968 when abortion was highly restricted by law. At that time, they referred women to private doctors in the U.S. and occasionally in foreign countries. Since legalization of abortion in 1973, their activities have slowly declined. Zero Population Growth was also formed in 1968 to stabilize population growth through educational, political, and legal means. Though it continues to be a very active political organization with over 300 chapters in the U.S., it no longer provides abortion referral services.

If you choose a nonprofit abortion referral agency, they will arrange your abortion for you free of charge, tell you where to go, what to do, and the cost of the abortion. To avoid delay in finding the safest and best place for your abortion — where the doctors are well-trained in abortion techniques — choose one of these dependable agencies. If, however, you do not have access to a referral agency or prefer to locate your own abortion facility, there are certain things you should look for when choosing an abortion center. (See the next section on Choosing an Abortion Center.)

☐ CHOOSING AN ABORTION CENTER

If you choose to locate your own facility, whether in a clinic, doctor's office, or hospital, there are certain things you should investigate *before* deciding upon a place for your abortion. (As a patient, you have the right to know in advance the details of the services offered.) Not every type of facility exists in every town, but most of them are located in larger cities. Hopefully, wherever you live, there will be at least one of these abortion facilities. If not, be sure to seek advice in your nearest city.

There are basically four types of abortion facilities: freestanding clinics; hospital outpatient clinics; doctor's offices; and hospital with overnight stay. All should meet the requirements in the following checklist.

Types of Centers

Freestanding Clinics. Most abortions are done in freestanding clinics: clinics "freestanding" from hospitals that specialize in less costly, early abortions. To work well, these clinics exclude women more than 12 weeks pregnant and women with medical or gynecologic problems.

Some of these freestanding clinics offer only abortions. Others are multi-service birth control centers that offer abortions in addition to contraception, sterilization, and general gynecology services. There are also a few feminist women's health centers that offer abortions as well as other gynecology services in an environment controlled and operated by women.

Hospital Outpatient Clinic. Many major cities nationwide have hospitals that provide first trimester abortions. Obviously, hospitals have the most complete emergency facilities. Unfortunately, not enough hospitals provide first trimester abortions.

Doctor's Office. Some private doctors perform vacuum aspiration in their office for women who are up to eight weeks pregnant. A few doctors perform vacuum aspirations and D and C's for women 7 to 12 weeks pregnant, though most doctors prefer to do these procedures in a hospital outpatient clinic. Unless the doctor has emergency backup services, is experienced in current abortion techniques, and meets the requirements in this checklist, choose another place for your abortion.

Hospital With Overnight Stay. This is often — but not always — required for second trimester abortions, especially saline and prostaglandin labor induction. Though a growing number of clinics now offer the option of sterilization (laparoscopy) with abortions — depending on where you live and your overall health status — hospitalization may be necessary. Women with the following medical conditions also require hospitalization: heart disease; blood clotting disease; moderate to severe anemia; kidney disease; or sickle-cell anemia.

Checklist

Whether you call or visit an abortion center, this checklist will help you locate a safe, high quality abortion center:

- First, you should know that as an abortion patient, you are entitled to the same rights as any other patient. (See Chapter 1, Patient Rights.) Furthermore, your needs for counseling, complete information, tenderness, and understanding may be even greater.

- Are you medically screened by telephone before your abortion appointment to make certain you are eligible?

- If you are having your abortion done in a clinic or hospital, is it licensed or accredited by the state or local health department? This is not a legal requirement and will not always guarantee good care.

- If you are having your abortion done in a doctor's office, is the doctor trained in obstetrics and gynecology and licensed to practice in the state? (You can call your local medical society for this information.) Is the doctor experienced in current abortion techniques, does he/she know how to manage its complications, and does he/she meet all the other requirements in this checklist?

- Is a positive pregnancy test required before abortion? This is important for several reasons. First, you may not be pregnant. Some women become so panicky when their period is late that they try to get an abortion when they are not even pregnant. Second, you should have a reliable pregnancy test done *before* the day of your abortion by a certified lab to reduce the chance of errors. Do not use a do-it-yourself test as a substitute for a test done by a medical laboratory. If you are traveling out-of-state for your abortion, be sure to have a positive pregnancy test before making any travel plans.

- Is the facility equipped to handle emergencies? Is it affiliated with a backup hospital less than ten minutes away?

- Does the facility offer the following counseling services: help you make a decision about your unwanted pregnancy and discuss alternatives (abortion, keep the baby, adoption, foster home); feelings about your partner; description of the abortion procedure; post-abortion instructions; birth control. Counseling, either individual or group, provides good emotional support.

- If you want an IUD, will the doctor insert one at the time of the abortion? (Many IUDs are inserted at this time.) Is it one of the few clinics that offer the option of sterilization with the abortion?
- Is a medical and laboratory workup done before your abortion? The medical workup should include: medical and gynecologic history; measurement of blood pressure; physical and pelvic exam; and testing and necessary treatment for gonorrhea and syphilis. You should also be questioned about your current medication usage and any allergies to anesthesia or antibiotics.

   The laboratory workup should include: Pap test; pregnancy test (if not already done); urine test; and blood test (hematocrit and Rh factor). Your hematocrit checks for the presence of anemia; your Rh factor measures if your blood is Rh-negative or Rh-positive. If you are Rh-negative, you should receive an anti-Rh gamma globulin shot (vaccine) within 72 hours after your abortion to prevent problems with future pregnancies. Most facilities provide this shot; those that don't will tell you where to get one.
- Do you have a choice of anesthesia? Anesthesia can be local (deadens the pain through an injection in or near the cervix) or general (makes you unconscious).
- Does it require written informed consent before abortion? Since the early 1970s, federal and state governments have legally required that before any medical procedure all patients be provided with an explanation of the treatment, its benefits, known risks, side effects, and a description of any alternatives that would be advantageous to the patient. Even after you sign this form, you can change your mind about having an abortion.
- Does your state require written consent from your parents (if you are under 18) or from your husband? Laws vary from state to state. Check with Planned Parenthood or another nonprofit agency to see what your legal rights are in your state.
- What is the method of payment? Does it require advance payment with a check or cash? Are you charged accord-

ing to your ability to pay? Does it accept health insurance or Medicaid (Welfare)? As of June 1977, Congress passed legislation ruling that states did not have to spend federal Medicaid funds for all abortions but that states could limit payment to so-called "necessary" or "therapeutic" abortions. As for now, policy varies greatly from state to state. This means that some states are not paying for any abortions; others only under "certain circumstances;" and a few states pay for abortions on request to Medicaid-eligible applicants. Call your local Medicaid office about the current regulations in your state.

- Is there a recovery area for postoperative rest, medical observation, and discharge by the physician?
- Does the facility give you instructions telling you what to expect after the abortion and a 24-hour phone number to call in case of any serious problems? Does it also make arrangements for follow-up including counseling on birth control?

□ **TYPES OF ABORTIONS**

MENSTRUAL REGULATION
WHEN: UP TO 6 WEEKS LMP
WHERE: A FEW CLINICS AND DOCTOR'S OFFICES

Menstrual regulation—vacuum aspiration of the uterus within 14 days after the late menstrual period—is a safe way to end a *suspected* pregnancy. To the great confusion of both the medical literature and general press, it currently goes under several names. It is widely known as menstrual regulation, and less commonly as endometrial aspiration, preemptive abortion, and interception of pregnancy. If used by women's self-help groups to avoid menstrual flow rather than end a suspected pregnancy, it is termed menstrual extraction.

Menstrual regulation is a simple, safe, inexpensive surgical procedure much like having an IUD inserted. Beforehand, most doctors inject local anesthesia on either side of the cervix to numb the cervix and uterus. Without cervical stretching (dilation), the doctor inserts a thin, soft, flexible tube through the cervix and into the uterus. This tube is attached to a source of suction (syringe, mechanical pump, or electrical pump) that sucks out the lining of the uterus normally shed during the menstrual period plus the embryo if you are pregnant. Menstrual regulation — which can cause brief abdominal cramps — takes a short time, usually five minutes. You can leave the office or clinic within 30 to 60 minutes.

Menstrual regulation offers a number of advantages to the woman with a suspected pregnancy. For one, it is a safe, easy, inexpensive procedure. Moreover, many women find the term "menstrual regulation" easier to accept than the word "abortion." And, if you have had intercourse and suspect you are pregnant, you don't have to wait to have a pregnancy test.

Yet there are some disadvantages to menstrual regulation. It is not 100 percent effective in ending pregnancy or in removing all the monthly lining of the uterus. About three percent of all women continue their pregnancy and require further treatment. Because of the small chance of continued pregnancy, be sure to have a pregnancy test and pelvic exam one to two weeks after menstrual regulation.

Also, menstrual regulation represents medical treatment without diagnosis. Because it does not require positive proof of pregnancy, a significant number of women are not pregnant at the time of the procedure. In fact, among women with a period one week late, 50 percent are not pregnant. Among women with a period two weeks late, 15 to 30 percent are not pregnant. Though a delay of one week reduces the number of menstrual regulations, a significant number of nonpregnant women still receive unnecessary surgery.

VERY EARLY ABORTION
WHEN: UP TO 7 TO 8 WEEKS LMP
WHERE: A FEW CLINICS AND DOCTOR'S OFFICES

Very early abortion—vacuum aspiration of the uterus within four weeks past the missed menstrual period—is a safe way to end a pregnancy. It is similar to menstrual regulation in every respect, except that it requires positive proof of pregnancy.

Clearly the need exists for an accurate and inexpensive test capable of detecting very early pregnancy. Currently available laboratory tests are not reliable until two weeks after the late menstrual period. Two new blood tests—radioimmunoassay and radioreceptorassay—have made pregnancy detection possible even before a missed period. Unfortunately, these tests are too expensive for general use in clinics and doctor's offices and—for this reason—are only available in well-equipped hospitals and medical centers. When available, they will eliminate unnecessarily performed menstrual regulations and allow all women the opportunity to obtain simple, safe, virtually trouble-free abortions before their missed period.

FIRST TRIMESTER ABORTION
WHEN: 7 THROUGH 12 WEEKS LMP
WHERE: CLINICS, DOCTOR'S OFFICES, HOSPITALS

Dilation and Suction Curettage

This procedure—also called vacuum suction, vacuum aspiration, uterine aspiration, or other similar terms—is newer than the D and C. It is currently used for 90 percent of all first trimester abortions and may replace the D and C entirely. Not only is it easier and safer—allowing many clinics and doctor's offices to use it—but it is swifter. Suction curettage, which can cause brief but strong abdominal cramps, usually takes only five minutes.

Using local anesthesia (rarely general), the doctor widens (dilates) the opening of your cervix with successively larger rods. In special situations, doctors widen the cervix beforehand with rods of dried seaweed. (More about that later.) Then, instead of scraping the walls of the uterus with a curette (D and C), the doctor inserts a thin, nonflexible tube through your cervix into the uterus. This tube is attached to a source of suction that vacuums out the contents of your pregnant uterus. The more advanced the pregnancy, the more suction curettage is required. Many doctors use a curette after suction curettage to make certain that the uterus is completely empty of its pregnant contents. The recovery time following this method is generally two hours of rest and medical observation.

Dilation and Curettage

Until introduction of suction curettage, dilation and curettage, — or D and C for short — was the standard way to treat all first trimester abortions. Now it is used only for 10 percent of all first trimester abortions.

In this procedure, successively larger rods are used to widen (dilate) the opening of the cervix. A curette, a spoon-shaped instrument, is introduced into the uterus; the lining of the uterus plus the fetus is scraped out. D and C — which can cause brief but strong abdominal cramps — takes a short time, usually 20 minutes.

Many hospitals and clinics now offer D and C's with local rather than general anesthesia, allowing you to leave the facility after one to two hours of rest and medical observation. Some hospitals and clinics in various parts of the country use general anesthesia and require several hours stay or an overnight stay following the operation. (The need for overnight stay and general anesthesia continues to be a subject of debate.) Not all women are able to take advantage of local anesthesia on an outpatient basis. If you have a history of medical or gynecologic conditions, doctors generally perform D and C's in the hospital and require an overnight stay.

SECOND TRIMESTER ABORTION
WHEN: 13 THROUGH 24 WEEKS LMP
WHERE: CLINICS, HOSPITALS

Second trimester abortions are far more difficult physically, emotionally, and financially than first trimester abortions. In fact, so much, that a first trimester abortion is seven times safer than a second trimester one.

Though about 90 percent of all women obtain first trimester abortions, about 10 percent delay seeking abortions until the second trimester. These include teenagers who hide their pregnancies from their parents; women having difficulty in resolving their conflicts about abortion; women without access to information on where to go; women with a drastic change in life situation (separation or death of partner, for example); women with medical problems; and women with menstrual irregularities at the time of menopause who are not even aware of being pregnant.

And there may be some further delay. You may have to wait out the "interim period" from the 13th through the 15th week of pregnancy. Injections into the amniotic sac (labor induction) cannot be done until a woman is about 16 weeks pregnant. This is because the uterus and amniotic fluid surrounding the fetus are not ready before that time. Occasionally, some abortion facilities do D and C's and suction curettages between the 13th and 15th week. Moreover, some doctors use dilation and evacuation through the 20th week of pregnancy.

During the interim period it is not uncommon for many women to become extremely anxious, change their minds, and decide to continue their pregnancy after all. Whatever your decision, you legally have the right to obtain an abortion through the second trimester of pregnancy. But, even though abortion law permits pregnancy termination until this time, it also gives doctors and the State the right to refuse late abortions. Many doctors exercise this right—especially between the 20th and 24th week—making it *very* difficult for women to obtain late second trimester abortions.

You should try to obtain a first trimester abortion. The earlier your abortion is performed, the fewer the risks, both physically and emotionally.

Saline Labor Induction

Before saline labor induction, or "salting-out," the doctor injects local anesthesia into your abdomen. A needle, inserted through the abdomen, uterus, and into the amniotic sac, removes some of the amniotic fluid that surrounds the fetus. Then a highly concentrated salt (saline) solution that kills the fetus is very slowly injected into the sac. Contractions of the uterus usually start in a short time. Within 10 to 30 hours, sometimes over 40 hours, labor begins. If labor-inducing drugs or dried seaweed are used, labor starts much earlier. Often doctors widen the cervix in advance with sterile rods of dried seaweed (*laminaria digitata*). If inserted into the cervical canal about 12 hours before labor induction, the *laminaria digitata*—by absorbing moisture from the cervix—slowly and painlessly stretch the cervix.

Labor is relatively painless until delivery, when vaginal pain similar to childbirth is often experienced. If the pain is severe, you can request a pain-reducing drug. Following labor, the fetus and placenta are expelled. If the placenta is not expelled one to two hours later, your doctor removes it manually or surgically to prevent complications.

Most hospitals have you remain in the hospital during the waiting period, making your hospital stay about two days. Others let you go home with instructions to return when contractions start. Though you do not run any physical risk by going home, it may be much more difficult emotionally. Of the two, staying in the hospital is preferable.

Before saline induction, you should be carefully screened

for medical problems. All women except those with the following medical conditions can receive this method: sickle-cell disease; heart disease; kidney disease; or hypertension.

Most doctors who perform saline labor induction find it a safe way to end a second trimester abortion. But complications can occur in some women. These include: hemorrhage; infection and/or fever; cervical tear; retained placenta. In rare instances, potentially serious complications can occur: blood clotting disorder; or injection of saline into the blood stream instead of the amniotic sac causing symptoms of headache, restlessness, finger numbness, body warmth and excessive thirst (hypernatremia). In extremely rare cases, hypernatremia can cause death.

Prostaglandin Labor Induction

In late 1973 the Food and Drug Administration approved use of a synthetic prostaglandin (fat-like substance naturally present in the body) for second trimester abortions. The prostaglandin technique is the same as saline. But it works by causing intense contractions of the uterus which expel the fetus and placenta.

Compared to saline, prostaglandin has some advantages. For one, labor starts several hours sooner. Moreover, even though women using this method may require a second injection, prostaglandin lacks the risk of developing blood clotting disease and hypernatremia. Yet there are some disadvantages to prostaglandin. Severe nausea, vomiting, and diarrhea are brief but common side effects. Other complications may include: hemorrhage; retained placenta; infection, chills, fever; asthma-like shortness of breath; or seizures. While these complications are uncommon, they do occur more often in women using prostaglandin than saline.

As with saline, you should be screened for medical problems. All women except those with the following medical conditions can use this method: pelvic inflammatory disease; history of convulsions; epilepsy; or asthma. Though doctors feel that women with sickle-cell disease, heart disease, or kidney disease can use prostaglandin, if you have one of these medical conditions, you should receive close medical supervision during the entire procedure.

Dilation and Evacuation

Occasionally, some abortion facilities use D and C and suction curettage between the 13th and 15th week; rarely after that. Though an increasing number of doctors now use dilation and evacuation after the 15th week, many don't, because they consider this method far riskier than labor induction. Since the early 1970s, however, several studies have shown that dilation and evacuation — contrary to popular belief — appears to be safer than saline labor induction through the 20th week. For now, further studies are needed to confirm the nature of these findings in addition to the long-term effects of this method before it can become a more widely accepted method of second trimester abortion.

Using either local or general anesthesia, the doctor widens (dilates) the opening of the cervix with successively larger rods. After dilation, the fetus and placenta are removed with forceps. To totally clean the uterus of its pregnant contents, doctors use a curette or suction curettage. Dilation and evacuation — which can cause brief but strong abdominal cramps — takes a short time, usually 30 minutes. Unlike labor induction, doctors perform it on a hospital outpatient basis, rather than in a hospital with overnight stay.

Hysterotomy and Hysterectomy

Until introduction of saline and prostaglandin labor induction, all second trimester abortions were surgically treated with hysterotomy or hysterectomy. Hysterotomy — often confused with hysterectomy — is like a cesarean section. The fetus is removed through an incision in the abdomen and uterus. Though this does not end fertility — unless a sterilization procedure is combined with it — hysterotomy usually limits future deliveries to cesarean section. Hysterectomy, on the contrary, is surgical removal of the uterus, which of course prevents future pregnancies.

Because these procedures are very costly and can be associated with serious complications, they are rarely used for second trimester abortions. Instead, they are reserved for the following reasons: women unable to use saline or prostaglandin labor induction; women with gynecologic problems requiring hysterectomy (for example, symptom-causing fibroids or endometriosis); and occasionally when another method fails.

☐ AFTER THE ABORTION

Aftercare Instructions

The abortion is over. Before you go home, you should receive written aftercare instructions telling you what to expect and what to do after the abortion. Your abortion facility should also give you a 24-hour phone number to call in case of emergencies after you return home. For your present and future health, be sure to follow these instructions:

- Take it easy for a few days. Get lots of rest. Though every woman's recovery time varies, most women resume their normal activities two to three days later.
- If your doctor prescribes pills to minimize bleeding and prevent infection, take them as prescribed. Try to eat well-balanced meals.
- You can expect bleeding for a few days, comparable to a normal menstrual period. However, if bleeding is more than a heavy menstrual flow or lasts longer than two weeks, get in touch with the clinic, doctor, or hospital that performed your abortion. Your normal period should start about four to six weeks after your abortion.
- You can also expect abdominal cramps for the first few

days. If they are excessive, get in touch with your abortion facility.

- If you develop a fever over 100 degrees, call your abortion facility promptly. Fever may be a sign of infection which requires immediate treatment.
- You should avoid douching, tampons, sexual intercourse, and baths (showers are okay) until your post-abortion checkup.
- If you have any unusual vaginal discharge, call your abortion facility.
- If you notice any other abnormal symptom after your abortion, call your clinic, hospital, or doctor promptly.
- See a gynecologist for a checkup two to three weeks after your abortion. This is very important for your present and future health.
- If you had your abortion because your method of birth control failed, you may wish to try another method to learn how to prevent future unplanned pregnancies. Some abortion facilities offer IUD insertion or even the option of sterilization at the time of abortion. Depending on your preference, others may give you a prescription for the birth control pill; if so, start taking your Pills right after the abortion. Or, if you prefer to use a diaphragm, wait until your post-abortion checkup to be fitted or refitted. If your post-abortion checkup is delayed past two to three weeks, use a combination of foam and condom until you see a gynecologist for advice about a reliable method of birth control.

Emotional Reactions

Your abortion is over and you are home. You are not receiving get-well cards, flowers, presents, lots of attention, and sympathy: the usual kind of comfort you receive from family and friends after an operation. Furthermore, you cannot talk about it at work or school, describing in detail just what happened. Unfortunately, when you have an abortion you are not apt to receive consolation. Given the moralistic atti-tudes that still exist, you may wish to keep your feelings to yourself. Or maybe your abortion was a deeply personal and private experience. Whatever your situation may be, you should talk to a close friend, your partner, an understanding relative, or join a rap group at your local women's center to let out your feelings, if you can.

No one knows how any woman will react to her abortion. Yet, after an abortion, many women feel in surprisingly good spirits. For most women, the first and strongest reaction is a sense of relief. A typical reaction might be: "While I hope I never have to go through another abortion, I can finally sleep nights again." While an abortion may bring out feelings of depression and sadness — a sense of loss or regret — these reactions are usually mild and temporary. A few women, however, experience emotional and sexual problems for some time after an abortion. If you continue to feel troubled, you may wish to ask your abortion facility for a referral to a therapist for support.

16

STILBESTROL EXPOSURE

Since 1971 diethylstilbestrol (called DES) has received an enormous amount of publicity, and rightfully so. Topics ranging from *DES to prevent miscarriage, DES as the morning-after pill,* and *DES as a food supplement for cattle and sheep* have caught the attention of medical journals as well as the media. But this chapter deals with only one of these issues: the use of DES to prevent miscarriage and treat the "high-risk" pregnancy. It turns out that after years of use, this medical practice was found to present health risks to some DES-exposed daughters and sons. And recent findings seem to have added a new cause of concern over the health risks to the mothers as well.

Whether you are a DES-exposed daughter or a mother who took DES during pregnancy, read on. Learn the facts and what to do.

☐ THE STILBESTROL PROBLEM

Diethylstilbestrol (stilbestrol, or DES as it is commonly called) was developed in 1938. When introduced to the market, it represented the first inexpensive, orally-effective synthetic estrogen in medicine. Its therapeutic uses were extensive: to suppress milk production after delivery; control menopausal symptoms; control irregular uterine bleeding; and control cancer of the prostate in men and cancer of the breast in postmenopausal women.

In the 1940s another use of DES became common: doctors used it to prevent miscarriage and treat the high-risk pregnancy. Though DES received approval for clinical use in 1940, doctors rarely used it at first. But by 1945 doctors frequently prescribed it to prevent miscarriage. It was actively used in the late 1940s and 1950s, with its use varying considerably from hospital to hospital in this country and abroad. Many doctors continued to use it less frequently, into the 1960s, even though an article appeared in the medical literature in the 1950s questioning the value of DES therapy for the high-risk pregnancy. In fact, this article concluded that there was *no* statistical evidence that DES effectively prevented miscarriage.

Finally, in 1971, the Food and Drug Administration (FDA) advised doctors against the use of DES and closely related drugs (such as dienestrol and hexestrol) for the treatment of high-risk pregnancies. This advice became necessary when researchers established an association between DES and clear cell adenocarcinoma, a very rare cancer of the vagina in adolescent daughters. Until 1971 this type of cancer was virtually unknown in women under 50.

Because of a 1971 ruling by the FDA, drug manufacturers now provide patient labeling with all DES prescriptions. This labeling states — among other things — who can and cannot use DES. No longer allowed for the prevention of miscarriage, here are the FDA's currently *approved* uses of DES:

> Estrogen replacement therapy for moderate to severe menopausal symptoms (hot flashes and vaginal dryness).
>
> Treatment of certain endocrine problems in younger women.
>
> To relieve the symptoms of certain advanced cases of cancer of the breast and prostate.
>
> Very shortly, the FDA will add osteoporosis (a bone disorder in postmenopausal women) to this list of approved uses.

Moreover, in February 1975, the FDA approved *limited* use of DES as a postcoital contraceptive (the so-called "morning-after" pill) for medical emergencies such as rape and incest. Despite this action, the FDA has not yet approved any marketing application for postcoital use of DES, even though DES is currently being used for that purpose, especially among college-age women. But the FDA is currently considering an application from one drug manufacturer for marketing DES as a postcoital contraceptive.

The FDA has placed special conditions on manufacturers wishing to market the drug as a postcoital agent. DES must be packaged in a 25 milligram dosage for this use. (The dosage of DES for postcoital contraception is 25 milligrams twice a day for five days.) The drug must also have specific labeling for doctors and patients. This means that anyone now using the morning-after pill is doing so without proper patient labeling. The labeling for all currently marketed DES (at five milligram dosage) specifically states that it should *not* be used as a postcoital contraceptive.

☐ PREGNANT MOTHERS WHO TOOK DES

Doctors prescribed DES to women who had complications of pregnancy or the so-called "high-risk" pregnancy. This generally included women with symptoms of vaginal bleeding, possible miscarriage, a history of prior miscarriage, diabetes, or hypertension. Many pregnant women who received DES say, "When I began spotting in early pregnancy, my doctor told me that I might lose my baby if I didn't take DES." Bleeding and possible miscarriage — which involve 10 percent to 20 percent of all pregnancies — generally occur in the first trimester or first twelve weeks of pregnancy, but can occur later. When prescribed, DES was given at the start of these symptoms.

According to research findings, the risk of developing DES conditions is related to the time of *in utero* exposure (fetal exposure to DES). Most genital conditions have occurred in daughters who were exposed before the 18th week of pregnancy. During this period the genital tract is forming in the embryo and it is extremely sensitive to agents causing birth defects. As for the amount of DES taken by the mother, it doesn't seem to bear any relationship to the risk of developing DES conditions.

☐ **HOW TO UNCOVER DES EXPOSURE**

If you suspect that you are a DES-exposed daughter or if you are a mother who took DES during one or more of your pregnancies, there are several ways to uncover DES exposure. First of all, DES was prescribed in the United States from the early 1940s to 1971. As of 1980, anyone currently between the ages of 9 and 40 years of age could have been exposed. Many, but not all doctors have sent notices to women who were given DES during pregnancy. If you have not received a notice, but suspect or know that you took DES, there are several ways to confirm DES history:

- Daughters who think they were exposed should question their mothers. But this is not always sufficient evidence. This is because not all mothers remember taking DES. Some women who claim they "Never took pills while pregnant," discover otherwise once their records are reviewed.
- Mothers who think they took DES should contact the doctor who treated them during pregnancy and ask for a review of their prenatal office record. If your doctor has retired or died, contact the hospital where your delivery occurred. The hospital may be able to tell you who has taken over the doctor's practice. If your prenatal office record is still available, request a review.
- Mothers should check the pharmacy where they purchased the DES. DES was prescribed in many different forms: pills, injections, suppositories, and vaginal creams. It was also sold under many different trade names. (See Table 12 for DES-type drugs that pregnant women may

TABLE 12. Trade Names of DES-Type Drugs

Amperone	Estrobene	Palestrol
AVC cream with	Estrobene DP.	Progravidium
Dienestrol	Estrosyn	Restrol
Benzestrol	Fonatol	Stil-Rol
Chlorotrianisene	Gynben	Stilbal
Comestrol	Gyneben	Stilbestrol
Cyren A.	Hexestrol	Stilbestronate
Cyren B.	Hexoestrol	Stilbetin
Delvinal	Hi-Bestrol	Stilbinol
DES	Menocrin	Stilboestroform
DesPlex	Meprane	Stilboestrol
Di-Erone	Mestilbol	Stilboestrol DP.
Diestryl	Methallenestril	Stilestrate
Dibestil	Metystil	Stilpalmitate
Dienestrol	Microest	Stilphostrol
Dienoestrol	Mikarol	Stilronate
Diethylstilbestrol	Mikarol forti	Stilrone
Dipalmitate	Milestrol	Stils
Diethylstilbestrol	Monomestrol	Synestrin
Diphosphate	Neo-Oestranol I	Synestrol
Diethylstilbestrol	Neo-Oestranol II	Synthoestrin
Dipropionate	Nulabort	Tace
Diethylstilbenediol	Oestrogenine	Teserene
Digestil	Oestromenin	Tylandril
Domestrol	Oestromon	Tylosterone
Estan	Orestol	Vallestril
Estilben	Pabestrol D.	Willestrol

have received.) Some pharmacies file prescriptions by family name and the pharmacist can easily locate the information. If this was not done, you may recall the month you started DES, or the month your first symptoms appeared. A search by the pharmacist of the prescriptions filled at the approximate date may provide the necessary information.

• Hospital birth records are occasionally helpful and are worth reviewing. In many states the patient (mother) has the legal right to review her medical record. Contact your hospital medical record department. You can request copies of your admission and delivery notes for a reasonable fee. DES, if prescribed, may be indicated on these notes. Be sure to get medical assistance if you have trouble understanding your record.

Perhaps you only *suspect* DES exposure but — due to un-located records — you aren't certain. If so, doctors still advise a screening exam. (More about that later.)

☐ EMOTIONAL REACTIONS

Discovery of DES exposure by both mothers and their daughters can be expected to create anxiety, fear about developing cancer, and for some others a sense of guilt. These are normal concerns that you should discuss with your doctor. Before the screening exam, both mothers and daughters should be well informed: you should ask about the DES problem; be told what to expect at the exam (a first experience for many daughters); and be allowed sufficient time for questions and answers. At the end of the exam, you and your doctor should discuss the findings; the risk of developing any kind of problems; treatment when necessary; and how often to schedule checkup exams. Any screening exam lacking these features is truly incomplete.

☐ SCREENING EXAM FOR EXPOSED DAUGHTERS

A gynecologic screening exam is a must for all DES-exposed daughters who have had their first menstrual period. If menstruation has not begun by age 14, an exam is still necessary. For younger daughters who have not menstruated, an exam is necessary only if symptoms such as vaginal bleeding or persistent discharge develop.

If you know or only suspect that you are a DES daughter, you can help your doctor by bringing any kind of information (mother's memory, prenatal office record, or hospital birth record, for example) to your first exam. This information will help your doctor carry out a more complete exam.

The exam should include careful visual and manual evaluation of the vagina and cervix. A Pap test should be taken. Though very effective in detecting cancer of the cervix, it is not always reliable for detecting DES-related cancers. The doctor should apply iodine solution (Schiller's test) to your vagina and cervix. If certain areas on your cervix or vagina appear abnormal, the doctor may remove a tiny amount of tissue (biopsy) for microscopic examination and diagnosis. Having a biopsy taken may be uncomfortable or, in some cases, slightly painful. Bleeding after biopsy may require the use of a vaginal tampon or feminine napkin. These diagnostic tests are vital since a routine gynecologic exam *cannot* diagnose many DES-related conditions.

A colposcope — a diagnostic instrument that simply magnifies the surface of the cervix and vagina — may be used for the exam. (See Chapter 18.) The colposcope helps gynecologists pinpoint suspicious areas for biopsy. Although the colposcope is helpful, it is not required and is not always available. Right now virtually every hospital associated with a medical school uses the colposcope. And yet, although present in many other well-equipped hospitals and in a large number of doctor's offices, colposcopes are not available for general use in all hospitals, clinics, and offices. If your doctor or clinic does not have access to a colposcope (ask about a referral), your doctor can still detect abnormal conditions by using iodine solution for biopsy.

After your screening exam, ask your doctor how often to schedule checkups. At the least, all DES-exposed daughters should have a checkup exam once a year. Most doctors, however, advise daughters with DES conditions to schedule checkups several times a year.

☐ **DES CONDITIONS**

DES-Exposed Daughters

Gynecologists frequently discover noncancerous conditions in DES-exposed daughters. While these conditions also occur in nonexposed women, they occur much more frequently in

DES-exposed daughters. These conditions are called cervical ectropion and vaginal adenosis. In these changes, tissue normally present in the cervical canal extends onto the cervix and into the vagina. Less-frequently found conditions include ridges in the vagina and on the cervix. So far, none of these conditions has been found to cause cancer, infertility, or sexual problems.

There have also been discoveries of some cancers. Women with cancer have ranged from 7 to 27 years of age at the time of diagnosis. On the average, most women are in their late teens. The vaginal and cervical cancers may be without symptoms, but usually cause vaginal bleeding, spotting, or discharge.

Mothers Who Took DES

As for the mothers who took DES during pregnancy, one medical center published a health survey in 1978 comparing DES users with a control group of non-DES users. Now, 25 years later, there were no health differences between the two groups. It turns out, however, that a slightly higher percentage of DES-users developed breast cancer than the non-DES users:

> Of 693 women who took DES, 32 (4.6 percent) developed breast cancer.
> Of 668 women who did not take DES, 21 (3.1 percent) developed breast cancer.

Moreover, after considering cancer of the breast and reproductive system together:

> Of 693 DES users, 48 (6.9 percent) developed cancer.
> Of 668 non-users, 31 (4.6 percent) developed cancer.

These statistics are not statistically significant, meaning that chance alone could easily account for the differences. Further research studies are needed to investigate what effect (if any) DES has on maternal health.

Right now doctors advise mothers who took DES to: have a yearly gynecologic exam with a Pap test and breast exam; practice monthly breast self-examination; and report promptly any abnormal breast findings to a doctor. Moreover, if you have a history of breast cancer or a strong family history of breast cancer, your doctor may recommend a yearly mammographic screening exam. Finally, unless you develop severe symptoms during menopause, think twice before taking estrogen replacement therapy. This is because the effects of estrogen replacement therapy on DES mothers are currently unknown.

DES-Exposed Sons

Since 1975 several medical centers have reported a small number of noncancerous genital conditions in DES-exposed sons. Though these conditions may also occur in nonexposed men, they occur much more frequently in exposed sons. These include: cysts on the epididymis (tube carrying sperm from the testes); small testes; undescended testes; and abnormalities such as low sperm counts. As a consequence of these findings, doctors now advise all DES-exposed sons to have a urologic screening exam.

☐ TREATMENT

The noncancerous conditions found in DES-exposed daughters don't generally require treatment. (If a doctor recommends treatment for one of these conditions, get a second medical opinion from a doctor experienced in handling DES conditions.) Most doctors, however, advise women with abnormal conditions to have regular checkups, possibly several times a year.

Women with cancer should receive their treatment from a gynecologist experienced in treating DES-exposed daughters. If your doctor is not experienced in this area, you should be referred to a doctor who is. The important thing is to get the best care you possibly can.

Treatment for cancer depends upon the amount of cancer

found at the diagnostic exam. Treatment generally involves surgery, radiation therapy, or a combination of the two. Most women are surgically-treated with radical hysterectomy. (See Chapter 18, Hysterectomy.) When it is necessary to remove the vagina, an artificial one can be constructed to replace it, making sexual intercourse possible after the vagina has healed; usually three months after surgery.

Cancer treatment varies from woman to woman. What is good for one woman may not be advisable for another. Your doctor makes a recommendation about treatment after consultation with several doctors. You may wish to have these recommendations discussed with your family and/or one of your close friends. The ultimate goal of any treatment plan is cure: elimination of all the cancer.

Regular checkups are a must for women with a history of cancer, so ask your doctor how often to schedule your exams. Of course, if you develop any abnormal symptoms between visits, call your doctor promptly. Generally, these exams include Pap tests and other laboratory tests. Checkups are essential, so be sure to keep your appointments. These exams enable doctors to provide treatment at the earliest possible time for any condition requiring further treatment.

☐ **DES EFFECT ON FERTILITY, SEXUALITY, AND CHOICE OF BIRTH CONTROL**

So far, researchers do not know if DES exposure has any kind of effect on fertility. Even so, cases of infertility, pregnancy outside the uterus, premature delivery, and cervical incompetence have been reported in DES-exposed daughters who have anatomic abnormalities of the uterus, cervix, and vagina. Right now, various researchers are trying to determine if these problems occur more frequently in DES-exposed daughters than nonexposed women.

Likewise, there is no evidence that DES exposure interferes with normal sexual activity or that certain methods of birth control are more helpful or harmful to DES-exposed daughters. Nevertheless, doctors tend to recommend methods such as the diaphragm over the birth control pill. This is because the long-term effects of the Pill on DES-exposed daughters are currently unknown.

☐ **DES-EXPOSED DAUGHTERS AND THE CANCER RISK**

Estimates show that several million daughters were exposed to DES during pregnancy. Out of this total, it seems that the risk of developing cancer is low. Overall, anywhere from 1 out of a 1,000 to 1 out of 10,000 DES-exposed daughters develop clear-cell adenocarcinoma of the vagina and cervix. Nearly 275 DES-related cancers have been reported to a cancer registry investigating this type of problem. Given the small number of cancers, it looks like the risk of developing cancer is rare for any DES-exposed daughter.

17

INFERTILITY

With frequent newspaper and television coverage about the newest advances in birth control and abortion, the subject of infertility may seem irrelevant and of minor concern. Yet an estimated 15 percent of all couples have trouble conceiving babies. Here is a sizable minority of American couples who have tried to have babies for a year or more, without success. In a woman, this means the inability to give birth to a live baby; in a man, the inability to impregnate a woman. For most infertile couples, the problem is failure of a sperm and an egg to unite. For others, it is failure of a fertilized egg to implant in the uterus or repeated miscarriages. In addition, infertility can occur when you try to have your first child (primary), or it can strike after one or more successful pregnancies (secondary).

Contrary to popular myths, infertility is *not*:

Just "A Woman's Condition." There are many reasons for infertility in *both* the man and the woman. After thorough medical evaluation, doctors uncover a medical problem about 80 percent to 90 percent of the time. Estimates show that a male problem exists about 40 percent of the time and a female problem about 60 percent. Moreover, about 20 percent of all infertility cases are the result of combined problems in both the man and the woman.

Usually Due to Emotional Factors. Infertility is not "all in your head." Anxiety and day-to-day emotional problems do not cause infertility, unless they interfere with normal sexual activity or disrupt ovulation or sperm production.

Incurable. The last decade has seen remarkable advances in the treatment of infertility. As new research and technology become available, the success rate for the treatment of infertility is improving. Today about 50 percent of all infertile couples can be helped to have a baby.

A Sexual Problem. Infertile couples are able to achieve the same sexual pleasures as other couples. Moreover, infertile couples are just as sexually appealing to each other as fertile couples are. An infertility workup can, however, be stressful to even the best sexual relationship.

Anyone's "Fault." Infertility is not anyone's fault. It is a *couple's* problem. Both partners must work together successfully to create a child.

Not so long ago little help could be offered to infertile couples. But today new medical and surgical treatment can help more than half of all couples have babies they want. Let's look at some of the ways of dealing with infertility right now.

☐ WHEN AND WHERE TO GET HELP

Failure to become pregnant within two to three months does not mean that you are infertile. In fact, research studies show that women who have intercourse regularly without birth control can expect to become pregnant as follows: 25 percent in the first month; 65 percent in six months; 80 percent in one year; 90 percent within 18 to 24 months. After that, pregnancy rarely occurs unless a doctor can detect and treat the cause of the infertility. If you have not conceived a baby after 12 to 18 months, consult a doctor. If you are over age 30, be sure to consult a doctor within six months, since the chances of pregnancy decline rapidly as you age, especially after age 30. And, if you or your partner have a fertility-related problem, consult a doctor as soon as you want to conceive.

Most couples go first to their family doctor or gynecologist, sometimes with discouraging results. If a routine exam and perhaps one or two basic tests fail to reveal the cause of the problem, doctors often say, "Go home and try again." But don't stick it out with a doctor who may not be experienced in infertility treatment.

Instead, ask your doctor for a referral—for both you and your partner—to a doctor specializing in infertility problems. If that doesn't work, call the gynecology department of your nearest medical school or hospital associated with a medical school; ask for the names of doctors specializing in infertility. Or, if you prefer, you can contact your local Planned Parenthood Center. If the Planned Parenthood in your area does not provide infertility services, they can refer you to a doctor or clinic specializing in this area. In addition, the American Fertility Society and Resolve—two national organizations concerned with infertility—can give you names of doctors nearest home or refer you to a nearby clinic. (See Readings and Resources.)

The number of doctors specializing in infertility is increasing rapidly. In addition, there are a number of infertility clinics and facilities in major hospitals and medical centers, in cities nationwide. These facilities combine a variety of medical talents to form a health care team, ranging from gynecologists and endocrinologists to psychiatrists and sex therapists. Since infertility is such a complex problem, doctors can treat it most quickly, efficiently, and economically—in the long run—in such places.

□ **DIAGNOSIS**

When it is time to consult a doctor for help, both you and your partner should go together. The once common belief that the woman was always to blame is false. It is well known that the man, the woman, or both partners are likely to have a problem requiring investigation. Diagnosis of the problem can only succeed with the cooperation of both the man and the woman. Though the sequence of diagnostic tests varies, it may include some or all of the following steps.

Medical and Sexual Histories

The first visit to a doctor starts with a series of questions covering you and your partner's general health, and family and personal history; questions about the pattern of your sex life; and questions about your menstrual history and previous method of birth control. It is important to answer these questions frankly, since your answers may have a direct bearing on why you and your partner have not conceived. In the course of history-taking, the doctor may be able to determine whether you and/or your partner have a problem affecting your fertility.

Common cause of infertility in the *woman* include the following:

> The Fallopian tubes may be closed, blocking the passage of sperm and preventing the union of a sperm and an egg. Gonorrhea, pelvic inflammatory disease, ruptured appendix, and endometriosis are leading causes of infertility. If not treated properly, these conditions can make pregnancy very difficult.
>
> The ovaries may be producing eggs very irregularly or not at all. (See Chapter 2, Physiology of the Menstrual Cycle.) Lack of ovulation may be due to a disorder of one of the endocrine glands, such as the ovaries, pituitary gland, or thyroid gland.
>
> Sperm in the vagina may be stopped from entering the opening of the uterus. If the cervical mucus is cloudy and thick at ovulation — rather than clear and watery — it can prevent sperm from swimming through the cervix to meet an egg in the Fallopian tube. Other factors such as a chronic cervical infection, polyps, or fibroids may also stop sperm at the cervix.

The fertilized egg may reach the uterus but be unable to attach itself to the wall and develop normally, thereby resulting in miscarriage. Most miscarriages, which affect about 15 percent of all pregnancies, occur during the first three months of pregnancy. One miscarriage does not mean you are infertile. If, however, you have two or more miscarriages in a row, consult a doctor about an infertility workup.

Physical or emotional stress may exist that also interferes with fertility. For example, anxiety and depression; long-term use of tranquilizers, the birth control pill, and alcohol; long-standing chronic illness; or even crash diets may affect fertility if they disrupt ovulation.

Common causes of infertility in the *man* include these problems:

The testes may be producing too few sperm or none at all. This can result from many factors. Having mumps complicated by inflammation of the testes after puberty is a common cause of abnormal sperm production. Other conditions may also include: lower sperm production; gonorrhea or prostatitis; viral diseases such as mononucleosis or hepatitis; testicular injury; varicose veins of the testes (varicocele), use of certain drugs; too-frequent intercourse (more than once a day for several days in a row); unusual rise in scrotal temperature (due to jockey shorts, athletic supporters, long hot baths, saunas, or occupational exposure to high temperatures).

The testes may be producing abnormal sperm which lack the ability to swim (low motility). This may be due to chronic prostatitis (inflammation of the prostate gland); rise in scrotal temperature; or, hormonal factors.

The tube carrying sperm from the testes to the penis may be blocked. Any past infection, such as improperly treated gonorrhea, may block sperm.

Physical or emotional stress may exist that also interferes with fertility. For example, anxiety and depression; impotence and premature ejaculation; chronic
illness; and excessive use of certain drugs and alcohol
may affect fertility, especially if any of these factors
interfere with normal sexual activity.

Common causes of *combined infertility in the couple* may
be any of those listed above. For example, mild endometriosis combined with low sperm production may be causing
the problem. Also, some shared problems may be:

Due to sperm antibodies or substances that fight off
sperm the way a vaccine immunizes against disease.
Some women develop antibodies to their partner's
sperm. It is also possible for a man to develop antibodies to his own sperm.

Occasionally, the problem is lack of knowledge. Some
couples don't know when the fertile days occur, or
how often to have intercourse during this time, or
what to do to increase the chances of pregnancy. By
taking your basal body temperature, it is possible to
find out your fertile days. (More about that later.)
Pregnancy is more likely to occur if you have intercourse on the day of ovulation plus the day before
and after. During these three days, don't have intercourse more than once a day if your partner has a
low sperm count. (A relatively infertile man's sperm
production decreases if he makes love too often.)
Moreover, if your partner's sperm are to remain in
close contact with your cervix, a good position for
intercourse is with your partner above and facing
you. In this position, your partner faces you while
you lie on your back with a folded pillow under your
hips to raise them. But, also continue making love
in the ways that give you pleasure so that your sex
life doesn't become routine and boring.

After intercourse, don't jump out of bed right away
and don't douche afterward. Also, don't use lubri-

cants such as K-Y jelly, vaseline, or creams. Use saliva or vegetable oil if you need lubrication since other lubricants and douching have a slight contraceptive effect.

Infertility Investigation

Frequently the medical and sexual histories in addition to general physical exams (including a pelvic exam for the woman and a urologic exam for the man) do not reveal anything unusual. When this happens, most doctors first turn their attention to the man, rather than the woman. This is because it is medically much easier to investigate the man's reproductive status than the woman's.

Infertility investigations vary among doctors. Commonly performed tests — whether done in a doctor's office, clinic, or hospital — may include the following:

Semen Analysis. This should be the first diagnostic step of the investigation. Also called a "sperm count," this test checks the fluid that the man ejaculates during sexual intercourse. After two to three days of avoiding sexual intercourse, the man collects by masturbation *all* of his ejaculate in a clean glass jar. Kept at room temperature, the semen should be delivered to the doctor's laboratory within one hour. To be certain of an accurate test, your partner should not collect his semen by withdrawal or in a condom, since the most active sperm may be lost. If your partner cannot, for personal or religious reasons, collect his semen by masturbation, the doctor can give him a special condom (not slightly spermicidal like other condoms) to be worn during intercourse.

Sometimes microscopic examination of the semen reveals a complete absence of sperm. Other times, it shows a low sperm count (less than 20 million sperm per milliliter); low motility or inability of sperm to swim (at least 50 percent of the sperm must swim for fertility); or abnormal sperm shapes and sizes (at least 60 percent of the sperm must be normal for fertility). Since many factors can affect a man's sperm count, your partner may need to repeat the test about a month later. If the sperm count is normal, your evaluation starts. If the semen analysis is abnormal, your partner should be referred to a urologist for further medical evaulation.

Basal Body Temperature. This is often the first diagnostic test to find out whether a woman is ovulating. By charting the body's temperature at rest, you can determine *if* you are ovulating, and if so, *when.* By taking your temperature every day for three to four menstrual cycles, it is possible to find out your fertile days or the time when pregnancy is most likely to occur. Though the basal body temperature is not an accurate indicator of the exact time of ovulation, most doctors suggest sexual intercourse on the expected day of ovulation, plus the day before and after.

Taking the basal body temperature is simple. (See Chapter 12, Temperature Method.) Even so, be sure to receive thorough instructions and temperature charts from your doctor.

Biopsy of the Endometrium. By removing a small piece of tissue from the lining of the uterus for microscopic examination, a doctor can tell if a woman is ovulating and, if so, whether the endometrium can maintain a fertilized egg. More specifically, this test shows if the hormones, estrogen and progesterone, are being produced in adequate amounts and at the right time in the menstrual cycle. Biopsy is usually done several days before the menstrual period. In this office procedure, the doctor gently widens the opening of the cervix and then inserts a small instrument which scrapes off or suctions out small pieces of the endometrium. Biopsy may cause mild, temporary cramping and slight vaginal bleeding.

Blood and Urine Tests. Well-equipped hospitals often use highly sensitive laboratory tests to obtain information about a woman's total hormonal status. In fact, doctors may use certain endocrine tests instead of the basal body temperature charts and biopsy of the endometrium.

Postcoital Test. This simple, painless test consists of collecting a sample of fluid (mucus) from the cervical canal for microscopic examination. By checking the cervical mucus several hours after sexual intercourse at the expected time of ovulation, a doctor can learn a number of things. Cervical mucus normally undergoes changes as ovulation nears. If sperm are seen swimming actively in normal numbers, the mucus is passable to sperm. If the cervical mucus shows no sperm or only dead ones, the mucus is not passable to sperm.

Even though the postcoital test is quite useful — if the first test is inconclusive or abnormal — most doctors repeat it several times in order to get a final result.

Rubin Test. Available since 1919, this simple office procedure checks for the passage of carbon dioxide through the Fallopian tubes. In this diagnostic test — best done before ovulation — a small rubber-tipped instrument is inserted through the cervical canal. By slowly releasing carbon dioxide into the uterus, gynecologists are able to tell if the tubes are open or blocked. If one or both tubes are open, the gas passes through the tubes into the abdominal cavity, often causing shoulder pain when you sit up. If both tubes are blocked, there is no passage of carbon dioxide.

Though the Rubin test is a simple office procedure, many doctors have turned their attention to a more reliable X-ray test, hysterosalpingography.

Hysterosalpingography. If the Rubin test is indefinite or shows an obstruction in the tubes, a special X-ray study of the uterus and Fallopian tubes is required. Usually done on an outpatient basis after the menstrual period but before ovulation, this test checks for the passage of dye through the uterus and tubes. In this test, a small amount of dye is slowly injected into the uterus, which then shows up on X-ray film of the uterus and tubes. If one or both Fallopian tubes are blocked, the X-ray pinpoints the location. If both tubes are open, the dye passes into the abdominal cavity and is harmlessly absorbed by the body.

Since this test may be somewhat painful and cause temporary abdominal cramps, your doctor may give you a pain medication or local anesthesia beforehand. Unless you are allergic to radiopaque dye, gynecologists prefer this test over the Rubin test because it is more accurate.

Laparoscopy and Culdoscopy. When all other diagnostic tests are inconclusive or fail to reveal any cause of infertility, culdoscopy or laparoscopy may provide answers. This is because these minor surgical procedures allow direct visualization of the uterus, ovaries, Fallopian tubes, and the pelvic cavity. Under anesthesia, a pencil-like viewing scope is inserted into a small incision in the upper vagina (culdoscopy) or, more commonly, in the abdomen (laparoscopy). Once the scope — equipped with lights and mirrors — is in place, a doctor can quickly check the pelvic organs for any abnormal signs.

□ TREATMENT

Infertility investigations reveal the cause of the problem in most couples. Not so long ago little help could be offered. Today new medical and surgical treatment can help over half of all infertile couples have babies. Treatment, of course, varies with the kind of problem. The common causes of infertility often receive the following treatment.

Women

The most treatment success comes with problems of ovulation. Recently the Food and Drug Administration approved use of two fertility drugs for inducing ovulation: Clomid and Pergonal. Basically, these drugs work by stimulating the pituitary gland to release its hormones more effectively (Clomid) or by actually providing the needed hormone (Pergonal). For greater effectiveness, Pergonal is always (Clomid sometimes) used with another hormone, human chorionic gonadotropin (HCG). The reason why a woman is not ovulating determines which fertility drug (if any) is for her. Fertility drugs, because they are so potent, must be used with caution. For this reason, they are usually prescribed in small doses for a few days. Regular pelvic exams (sometimes blood and urine tests) are also necessary. Both drugs do, however, have a tendency to cause multiple pregnancies. Because these drugs stimulate the ovaries to release more than one egg, about 10 percent to 20 percent of all women taking these drugs have multiple pregnancies (usually twins). Not every woman who takes fertility drugs becomes pregnant. Of about 80 percent to 90 percent who ovulate after several cycles of treatment, about 50 percent finally give birth to healthy babies. Women who do not ovulate after treatment may possibly be helped with surgery. Removal of a wedge of tissue from both ovaries (ovarian wedge resection) may bring back ovulation for certain problems.

Cervical problems also respond well to treatment. Infections such as chronic cervicitis can usually be cleared up with antibiotics or cryosurgery. For women with thick cervical mucus (not passable to sperm), very small doses of estrogen before ovulation may stimulate a greater output of normal cervical mucus. In other cases, having your partner's sperm placed past your cervix is a quick, effective office procedure. If the cervix or uterus is blocked with polyps or minor adhesions, a D and C may be done.

Until recently endometriosis required surgical treatment. Now this problem can very often be controlled with high doses of hormone therapy over a period of about six to twelve months. In this condition, bits of tissue from the endometrium become scattered throughout the pelvic cavity. (See Chapter 5.) Often these stray pieces of tissue attach themselves to the tubes and ovaries, making pregnancy very difficult. Hormone therapy works by actually shrinking up these bits of endometrial tissue. While doctors prescribe various types of hormone therapy, combination birth control pills are currently the most popular. Yet a new type of hormone therapy, danazol (Danocrine), may challenge their popularity. While both types of therapy essentially work by preventing ovulation and menstrual periods, danazol definitely seems to be more effective in clearing up endometriosis.

Whether danazol will replace the combination pills entirely remains to be seen. Until all the results of ongoing clinical studies are in, danazol is only being used in selected cases.

Sometimes damage to the Fallopian tubes (from advanced endometriosis or severe pelvic infection, for example) is so great that no amount of hormone therapy helps. Here surgery is necessary. Endometriosis and scar tissue on the ovaries, uterus, tubes, and any other affected organs can be removed. If the uterus is tied down with scar tissue, it can be freed up and re-suspended in a normal position. Lastly, to restore the normal function of the tubes, scar tissue around the tubes can be removed. Temporary hormone therapy after surgery is usually necessary to prevent future flare-ups. As for the success rate of surgical treatment, it does vary greatly from woman to woman.

Men

Treatment for male infertility does not have the same success rate as treatment for female infertility. In cases of low sperm counts with good motility, a number of approaches are possible. Exercise, proper diet, cutting back on alcohol, tobacco, and drugs along with adequate rest and relaxation may improve sperm production, at least in some men. Since wearing tight-fitting jockey shorts or athletic supporters for long periods of time can lower sperm counts, a switch to boxer shorts may help. If the tube carrying sperm from the testes to the penis is blocked or a varicocele is present, minor surgery is often helpful for this problem. Right now there is no drug that really works to improve sperm count or quality, though research in this area continues.

Artificial insemination, another procedure for achieving pregnancy, is less complicated than it sounds. The doctor simply takes the man's sperm (obtained by masturbation) and introduces them — during the woman's fertile period — into the vagina with a syringe. This method is generally reserved for men who have normal sperm counts and motility but who are unable to ejaculate within their partner's vagina.

If the problem is one of low sperm count, concentrating and deep freezing several ejaculations together to achieve a higher sperm count is currently being tried; so far, without much success.

If the woman is fertile but the man is not, still another approach — though socially, legally, and medically controversial — is the use of sperm from an anonymous donor. Doctors who specialize in this technique should screen both the sperm donor and prospective infertile couple very carefully. The donor is known only to your doctor who selects a man with good health and heredity and with physical and blood characteristics similar to those of your partner. Not only will the donor's identity remain unknown, but doctors strongly advise infertile couples not to inform their friends and relatives of their plans: on the grounds that the truth might later become known to the child. If pregnancy occurs, doctors frequently refer their women patients to an obstetrician who knows nothing about the artificial insemination. At delivery, your partner's name appears on the birth certificate as the father. Though used successfully by thousands of couples yearly, artificial insemination from an anonymous donor can be a difficult choice for many couples.

☐ EMOTIONS AND ALTERNATIVES

Most, if not all, couples who learn they can't have children experience a variety of feelings. The first and most common reaction is usually one of surprise and anger. Next may come painful feelings of sadness, emptiness, depression, and maybe questions about manhood or womanhood. This can be a terrible period to go through. While most couples eventually resolve their feelings, grieving can last a long time. The important thing is to express your feelings to each other, rather than hiding them inside. You may also wish to join a local support group of other infertile couples to let your feelings out, if you can. (See Readings and Resources.)

Alternatives worth exploring do exist. Adoption, satisfactory for many couples, is the traditional alternative. Until the 1970s, adoption of a healthy baby of one's own race was relatively easy. But today, abortion legislation, birth control, and the fact that over 70 percent of all single mothers now keep their babies, means that there are very few babies available for adoption. In short, babies for adoption are generally obtained with difficulty and often great expense through private sources, rather than through adoption agencies. But children of all races, children over six, sibling groups, and children with psychological or medical problems are available for adoption in every state. Currently, one of the most popular (yet increasingly controversial) sources of young, healthy babies is through international adoption is some foreign countries.

The adoption situation varies across the country. If you are unsuccessful with your local adoption resources, you may wish to contact Resolve, a national organization for counseling and help. (See Readings and Resources.)

18

SURGERY

When we hear the words surgery or operation, we think first of a cutting procedure and then of the financial expenses. Then — if we have heard or read about it — we think about second opinions, Board-certification, checking out a surgeon's qualifications, and so forth. The array of issues is confusing, indeed. It is even more confusing when a doctor recommends surgery. If this is your situation, consider these issues in relation to your personal needs. But realize also that delaying *necessary* surgery for too long can be hazardous to your health.

Gynecologic surgeons — as do other professionals — vary greatly in education, training, integrity, and compassion. Moreover, some doctors tend to be more conservative than others about recommending surgery. Others are more inclined to operate than use nonsurgical treatment. Even though it is easy to check out a doctor's credentials — such as where his/her medical degree was received, whether he/she is state-licensed or certified in a specialty, whether a member of prestigious surgical organizations, or published in professional journals — everyone goes about choosing a doctor in a different way.

Some women may already have a gynecologist who can perform their surgery. If your gynecologist is not experienced in treating your problem surgically, you should be referred to a doctor who is. Other women prefer to leave the choice up to their family doctor or internist. Still others rely heavily on the recommendations of friends and relatives who have undergone surgery. For example, "Dr. Jones took such good care of me when I had my surgery that I wouldn't think of going to anyone else." A statement like that from someone you know well could be the factor you rely on most.

Certainly for many women all of the above are the time-honored ways to choose a surgeon. Some of the best ways for you to select good surgical care are to:

- Ask plenty of questions about the reasons for any type of recommended surgery, especially major surgery like hysterectomy. Also, ask about all alternative types of treatment open to you. Other questions to ask could include: what will happen if you don't have surgery and what will happen if you wait and have it later?

  Make sure you have confidence in your surgeon.
- If you don't receive adequate answers to your questions, get a second surgical opinion about the necessity of any recommended major surgery from a Board-certified gynecologist. Your county or state medical society can give you names of qualified doctors able to tell you if your surgery is necessary. Almost all insurance companies pay for second opinions.

  Since early 1977 Medicaid (Welfare) has operated a Second Surgical Opinion Program. Right now this is currently mandatory only in Massachusetts. Other states, however, are working on optional programs that clearly express the concern of unnecessarily-performed surgery. This means that before nonemergency hysterectomy, Massachusetts women must get a second opinion about the necessity of their hysterectomy before Medicaid will pay for surgical expenses. Seven other surgical procedures, in addition to hysterectomy, also require a second opinion.
- For your surgery, choose a Board-certified gynecologist: a doctor least likely to give you bad advice. (See Chapter 1, Doctors.) Doctors who are Board-certified in obstetrics and gynecology have passed both written and oral examinations that require established levels of knowledge and standards of practice. One of the things that the American Board of Obstetrics and Gynecology tries to do is control unnecessary surgery. Your county or state medical society in addition to the *Directory of Medical*

Specialists can provide you with this information. The *Directory*, available at most public libraries, also provides information about a doctor's educational and professional background. (See Readings and Resources.)

It is essential to check out a doctor's credentials ahead of time. Believe it or not, 35 percent to 40 percent of all gynecologists are not certified by the American Board of Obstetrics and Gynecology: a statistic comparable with other surgical specialties. Fortunately, noncertified surgeons tend to do fewer and simpler operations than certified surgeons.

- Also, make sure to choose a gynecologist and not a general surgeon or general practitioner for your surgery. While all of these doctors receive training in surgery (general practitioners receive *very* little), only gynecologists receive specialty training in gynecologic surgery. For this reason, gynecologists are better qualified to perform any kind of gynecologic surgery.
- Hospitals where surgery is performed are not equal. (See Chapter 1, Hospitals.) Some are small and equipped only to handle simple surgery. Others are large and offer a dazzling array of sophisticated surgical services. Between these extremes are a variety of other hospitals where most surgery is performed daily. No matter what type of hospital you enter, make sure it is approved by the Joint Commission on Accreditation of Hospitals. You can check out a hospital's accreditation by asking your doctor or the hospital's administrative office. Since hospital standards do not have to be especially high to receive accreditation, you should avoid nonaccredited hospitals. By the way, about one out of four hospitals is not accredited.

☐ HYSTERECTOMY

Hysterectomy (removal of the uterus) is a fairly routine major surgical procedure. Why then is it the target of public criticism and the focus of medical controversy? Most importantly, hysterectomy is currently one of the most overused and costly surgical procedures, not without medical risks. In fact, current data disclose that it is one of the top four surgical procedures:

Vaginal delivery.
D and C.
Hysterectomy.
Tonsillectomy.

Not only is hysterectomy the second most frequently performed procedure in gynecology, but for every four deliveries in obstetrics, one hysterectomy is performed in gynecology. According to 1977 estimates from the National Center for Health Statistics, surgeons performed 705,000 hysterectomies. No other type of major operation is performed as frequently as hysterectomy. Moreover, if current rates continue to climb, statisticians predict that one-half of all U.S. women will undergo hysterectomy by age 65.

How many women actually have unnecessary hysterectomies? While surgeons perform hysterectomies for a wide array of problems ranging in severity from cancer to contraception, exact national statistics on the reason for doing hysterectomy do not exist. What does exist, however, is a commonly-held rationale, published in 1969 by an American gynecologist: "The uterus has but one function: reproduction. After the last planned pregnancy, the uterus becomes a useless, bleeding, symptom-producing, potentially cancer-bearing organ and therefore should be removed." An extreme position, but not uncommon. Unfortunately, such an argument is richer in financial benefits and surgical complications than having any real basis in fact.

Numerous books and articles have been published about unnecessary surgery, especially hysterectomy. You can avoid being victimized by this problem by becoming aware of the standard reasons for hysterectomy. While there are no hard and fast rules, the following problems *may* require hysterectomy:

Cancer and *some* precancerous conditions of the cervix, endometrium, ovaries, Fallopian tubes, and vagina.

Fibroids that cause pain, bleeding, or very large abdominal masses. If you want to have more children, see the discussion about myomectomy in Chapter 5, Fibroids. (Myomectomy removes the fibroids only and leaves the uterus.)

Endometriosis that causes pain, bleeding, or very large abdominal masses and is not treatable with hormones.

Severe abnormal uterine bleeding not treatable with hormones or D and C.

Advanced infections or diseases of the ovaries or tubes.

Advanced pelvic inflammatory disease; septic abortion not treatable with D and C and antibiotics.

Prolapse of the uterus, causing discomfort and pressure on the bladder or bowel, for example.

Life-threatening complication of delivery.

For abortion, when a standard method fails. (This is rarely necessary.)

For women *desiring* sterilization who also have one of the above gynecologic problems.

Until recently, hysterectomy was the most common method of sterilization. According to estimates, sterilization is still a major reason for hysterectomy in women under age 40. Yet hysterectomy for contraception alone represents unnecessary surgery. (See Chapter 14 for currently acceptable methods of sterilization.)

For whatever reason a doctor recommends hysterectomy, you, as a patient, have the right to be well-informed by your doctor. (See Chapter 1, Patient Rights.) Before surgery, the doctor should discuss various issues with you, your family, and/or one of your close friends. Your doctor should explain the reasons for recommending hysterectomy in relation to your existing problem. In addition, you and your doctor should discuss the risks, benefits, and side effects of hysterectomy, in addition to any alternative treatment that exists for you. As a patient, you have the right to complete and current information concerning your diagnosis, treatment, and prognosis. Make sure you understand what your doctor is saying. If you don't, say so.

The Hysterectomy Operation

Though policy varies from hospital to hospital, most women enter the hospital a day or two before surgery. During this preoperative period, you will see your own doctor, maybe a few other doctors, and some nurses. If you enter a teaching hospital — a hospital associated with a medical school — you may also see interns and residents (doctors in training) in addition to medical and nursing students. All of these professionals and students work with and under the direction of your own doctor.

Since surgery and anesthesia produce changes in the body, your medical team will want to know all about your current health status to plan the best and safest care for you. Before hysterectomy, you will receive a physical exam plus a series of tests to make certain that you are physically ready for surgery. These diagnostic tests usually include: blood and urine tests; a chest X-ray; and frequently an electrocardiogram (record of the heart's activity). Other tests may include: an X-ray of the kidneys (intravenous pyelogram); X-ray of the bowels (barium enema); exam of the bladder (cystoscopy); and rectum (proctoscopy). Before cancer surgery, other similar, but more specialized tests may also be necessary.

In addition to laboratory tests, a complete medical history of your past and present illnesses is important. Be thorough and accurate in relating your medical history. The day or evening before surgery, an anesthesiologist will also ask you about your medical history to see if you have any problem likely to interfere with your anesthesia. You will be asked about: your past experience with surgery; known allergy to a specific anesthetic agent or antibiotic; your current medication usage; and your history of respiratory problems. Depending on your situation, your anesthesiologist will choose general or regional anesthesia. General anesthesia makes you unconscious; regional anesthesia affects only your pelvic area. Before either type, you will receive a premedication that puts you into a drowsy state or complete sleep.

If you smoke, it is essential that you severely limit or stop smoking for several weeks before surgery. Smoking puts surgical patients "at risk" for developing respiratory problems in addition to other complications after surgery. If you use estrogens (birth control pills or estrogen replacement therapy) you should stop using them at least four weeks before surgery, if this is possible. This is because estrogens put surgical patients "at risk" for developing blood clotting disorders. Finally, if you are extremely overweight, your surgeon may delay your operation until you lose some weight. Obesity, like smoking and estrogens, increases the risk of developing complications.

Depending on the reason for your hysterectomy, your surgeon will remove your uterus in one of two ways: through the abdomen or the vagina. In *abdominal hysterectomy* — the most common type of hysterectomy — the uterus including the cervix is removed through a six to eight inch incision in the lower abdomen. Though surgeons haven't always removed the cervix (*subtotal hysterectomy*), better surgical techniques have made *total abdominal hysterectomy* — removal of both the uterus and cervix — the rule. In *radical hysterectomy*, the uterus, cervix, surrounding tissues, upper vagina, and usually the pelvic lymph nodes are removed. Radical hysterectomy is a form of cancer surgery that is almost always performed by a surgeon trained in gynecologic cancer surgery. In all abdominal hysterectomies, the scar, which will be below the navel, may be horizontal or vertical. In *vaginal hysterectomy*, often reserved for uterine prolapse, the uterus and cervix are removed through the vagina.

Hysterectomy does not lower estrogen levels unless the ovaries are removed (*oophorectomy*). This means that if your ovaries are not removed, you will continue to ovulate but will never have another menstrual period nor be able to get pregnant. Unless ovarian disease is present, surgeons don't usually remove the ovaries in younger women. Even if the ovaries are normal in women in their late thirties and early forties, some surgeons routinely remove them; others leave them in. Why surgeons move one way or the other continues to be a debatable issue. So make sure you know what your surgeon plans to do about your ovaries before hysterectomy.

Hysterectomy does not bring about menopausal symptoms

unless *both* ovaries are removed. Even removal of one ovary does not cause menopausal symptoms, since the remaining ovary continues to produce enough estrogens. If you are over age 50, when the risk of developing ovarian disease and cancer increases, your surgeon — to prevent problems that might require further surgery — will most likely remove both ovaries. Removal of both ovaries and Fallopian tubes (done for technical reasons) is called *bilateral salpingo-oophorectomy*. If you have not gone through your natural menopause, but the surgeon removes both of your ovaries, you will most likely go through a "surgical menopause." This means that hot flashes and vaginal dryness — symptoms related to decreased levels of estrogens — may develop a week or so after surgery. If you develop hot flashes and vaginal dryness, ask your doctor about estrogen replacement therapy for relief of your symptoms. (See Chapter 21, Estrogen Replacement Therapy.) If you choose to use estrogens, be sure to request the lowest effective dose for the shortest possible time.

After Hysterectomy

For the first day or so after surgery, you will not eat solid foods. Instead, you will receive sugar and usually salt solution intravenously for nourishment. Usually a slim tube (catheter) extends out of the urethra (channel that carries urine from the bladder). This tube keeps the bladder drained of urine during a time when it is difficult, if not impossible, to urinate without assistance. All of these tubes are rarely needed for more than several days.

Pain after any kind of surgery is common. The incision usually causes a moderate amount of pain on the first day or two. After the first week, most of the discomfort goes away. On the third or fourth day after surgery, temporary abdominal gas pains develop as the stomach gets used to digesting food again. After that, abdominal pain subsides. During your stay in the hospital, it is possible to request pain medications as you need them. After you go home, your doctor will prescribe medications if you continue to need them.

To speed recovery and minimize postoperative complications, such as inflammation of leg veins caused by poor circulation (phlebitis) and respiratory problems, your doctor will encourage moderate activity soon after surgery. The first day after surgery, a nurse will get you up and help you walk a few steps. While difficult at first, strength increases with each successive period out of bed. After the first week, most women are well enough to be discharged from the hospital to continue recovery at home.

Healing takes time. Stitches, if they require removal, are usually removed before you leave the hospital. At first, the scar will be red and swollen. As it heals, it will approach your skin color. Within a few weeks, just a line of scar tissue remains.

Prior to discharge from the hospital your doctor should give you at-home instructions regarding what side effects to expect. Some of the more common side effects of hysterectomy are bladder and wound infections (treatable with antibiotics) in addition to difficulty urinating. Other things to discuss include: care of your incision, bathing, douching, diet, exercises, and sexual activity. If you develop any abnormal symptoms after you leave the hospital, call your doctor promptly. Otherwise, mention any minor problems at your postoperative checkup. Whether or not your cervix is removed, checkups with a Pap test are still important. This is especially true for women with a history of cervical cancer. How often you need to have checkups varies from woman to woman. So ask your doctor how often to schedule your exams.

After surgery, it takes several weeks for complete healing and for all of the pain to go away. You will probably have a little discharge and slight vaginal bleeding for a few weeks. If you develop heavy bleeding, call your doctor, since minor treatment, such as a few stitches, may be necessary. After the stitches are removed (five to seven days after surgery), you can resume bathing or showering, but check with your doctor beforehand. Also, avoid douching unless directed by your doctor.

Your diet should contain foods rich in protein such as eggs, fish, meat, and milk; drink lots of fluids to help prevent bladder infections; and eat fresh fruits and vegetables to help restore bowel function and prevent constipation. During this inactive period, it is easy to gain weight. Any increase in weight is not due to removal of the uterus and/or ovaries but to eating more and exercising less. For this reason, limit your intake of carbohydrates (starches) and fats.

The return of physical strength is slow but steady, and most women are able to resume their normal activities four to six weeks after their hysterectomy. But to feel normally energetic may take up to six to twelve months. During this recovery period, gradually resume your activities. For the first two weeks at home, be sure to rest more than usual by getting out of bed late, into bed early, and napping for an hour in the afternoon. Over the next two weeks, it is possible to start light activities at home and outdoor walks. Heavy lifting, energetic activities, and a few simple exercises to retone the muscles should wait four to six weeks, at least. Women vary as to when they are ready to resume their former activities. Basically, women with sedentary jobs can usually return to work in about six to eight weeks.

As for sexual activity, your surgeon should discuss what to expect *before* hysterectomy. This discussion should include both you and your sexual partner. Discussing when you can resume sexual activity, any changes in sexual arousal that may occur, in addition to counseling on different sexual techniques, can go a long way to prevent future problems. In general, you should not have intercourse until the vagina is completely healed. This usually takes six to eight weeks after abdominal or vaginal hysterectomy and three months after radical hysterectomy. Only your doctor, however, can confirm complete healing at your postoperative checkup. During this interim period, you and your partner can substitute alternative methods for vaginal intercourse. After this time, gentle sexual intercourse (without deep thrusting) is usually possible. Initially your abdomen may be sensitive. It may take up to six months before normal sexual activity can be enjoyed, not merely tolerated.

After recovery, many women — freed from menstrual

periods, fears of pregnancy, and prehysterectomy symptoms — often find sexual fulfillment during this time. Lovemaking often becomes more relaxed and spontaneous. On the contrary, some women may recoil from sexual activity due to painful intercourse. Unless your ovaries were also removed, hysterectomy should not cause menopausal symptoms of painful intercourse and vaginal dryness. Consult your doctor if you continue to have painful intercourse or a reduction in sexual arousal after your recovery period. If you have not gone through your natural menopause and your ovaries were removed, you may well go through a "surgical menopause." This means that hot flashes and vaginal dryness — symptoms related to decreased levels of estrogens — may develop a week or so after surgery. If this becomes a problem for you, ask your doctor about estrogen replacement therapy for relief of your symptoms. If you choose not to take estrogens, K-Y jelly (available at drugstores without a prescription) is often an effective vaginal lubricant.

A wide variety of attitudes toward hysterectomy exist. Contrary to popular belief, hysterectomy — with or without removal of the ovaries — should not change you as a person. It will not make you less of a woman, cause premature aging, put an end to your sex life, or make you less attractive or desirable. Furthermore, hysterectomy will not deprive you of your energy after recovery, make you grow unwanted hair, or "clean you all out." Even so, these are normal concerns that you should discuss with your doctor before hysterectomy. Often review of the pelvic anatomy, along with a discussion of what is and is not being removed in addition to what the uterus means to you, can go a long way to prevent future problems.

Emotional changes after hysterectomy vary from woman to woman. A few days after surgery, many women feel weepy, sensitive, depressed, and let down. These feelings — quite common following any kind of major surgery — usually last a few days, sometimes longer. Within a month or so, most women feel like themselves again. While hysterectomy may bring about emotional stress, social factors as much as loss of reproductive ability may also do this.

Between the ages 40 and 50—when most women undergo hysterectomy—a woman is likely to lose her father and later her mother; if married, her children may leave home for college or marriage. If her husband is a failure she has to face this realization; if he is successful, he is frequently away from home. For the woman who has no family, hysterectomy marks the end of any childbearing possibility. And the woman who has not met her career aspirations has to face this realization also. All of these losses are real and, to varying extents, distressing to many women. Most women are able to deal with their hysterectomies and other social changes by talking things over with a close friend or sympathetic husband. Some women may need help from a therapist. If you need emotional support at this time, you may wish to ask your doctor for a referral to a therapist.

☐ D AND C

The most frequently performed operation in gynecology is the D and C, short for dilation and curettage. In this minor 20 minute procedure, successively larger rods are used to widen (dilate) the opening to the cervix. A curette, a spoon-shaped instrument, is then introduced into the uterus. The lining of the uterus, which is only loosely attached, is scraped out. All of this material is then sent to a medical laboratory for microscopic examination and medical diagnosis. If the pathology report reveals something abnormal, your doctor will contact you about further diagnostic tests and/or treatment.

Gynecologists can learn a number of things from a D and C and, in general, use it for any of the following reasons:

> Diagnose abnormal bleeding during or between menstrual periods if no cause for bleeding has been found at the office visit. Usually, a menstrual hormone disorder—such as failure to ovulate every month—is the problem; less often, polyps; and far less frequently, cancer of the uterus.

If a diagnostic D and C reveals a hormone disorder or polyps, the diagnostic D and C often serves as treatment.

To end first trimester pregnancies. Though 90 percent of all abortions are done with suction curettage, 10 percent are still done with D and C.

To treat incomplete miscarriage by removing retained fetal remnants.

To remove placental tissue left in the uterus after a normal full-term delivery.

To treat narrowing of the cervical canal (stenosis).

In addition, gynecologists often routinely perform a D and C before most gynecologic operations.

Most women undergoing D and C enter the hospital early in the morning for a few preoperative tests and leave the hospital several hours after postoperative rest and medical observation. To enable thorough manual examination of the reproductive organs — something that is not possible in conscious women — gynecologists prefer general rather than regional anesthesia during D and C.

Though D and C is generally without side effects, you may have a slight reddish-brown vaginal discharge several days after surgery. If you develop heavy vaginal bleeding, fever, or abdominal pain after surgery, call your doctor promptly.

☐ **COLPOSCOPY AND BIOPSY**

The colposcope — a diagnostic instrument that simply magnifies the surface of the cervix and vagina — didn't gain prominent acceptance among U.S. gynecologists until the early 1970s. During its early years of use, many gynecologists placed it in competition with the Pap test for early cervical cancer detection. Invariably, the Pap test was far less expensive and considerably easier for the gynecologist to learn about and use.

Colposcopy has found its place, though. Right now the Pap test is still the best way to *screen* all women for early abnormal cervical conditions. But gynecologists use the colposcope to investigate further certain groups of women. When available, colposcopy is very valuable in the following situations:

> Pap test suggestive of dysplasia or a more severe condition.
>
> Examination of stilbestrol-exposed daughters.
>
> Because colposcopy helps identify abnormal areas on the cervix and vagina, it minimizes the need for biopsy and cervical conization. By doing this, it reduces the number of unnecessarily performed biopsies and conizations. In about 20 percent of all women, the colposcope is not capable of examining certain regions of the cervical canal. When this happens, conization is necessary. (More about that later.) This means that colposcopy eliminates the need for conization in about 80 percent of all women with a Pap test suggestive of dysplasia or a more severe condition.

Colposcopy is a simple, painless, complication-free office procedure that takes about 15 minutes. The exam goes as follows: to see your cervix and vagina, the doctor inserts a speculum into your vagina. If the colposcope pinpoints suspicious areas on the cervix or vagina, your doctor may remove a tiny amount of tissue (*biopsy*). Having a biopsy taken may be uncomfortable and, in some cases, slightly painful. Vaginal bleeding after biospy may require the use of a vaginal tampon or feminine napkin. Biopsy material is then sent to a medical laboratory for microscopic examination and diagnosis. If the pathology report reveals something abnormal, your doctor will contact you about further diagnostic tests and/or treatment.

Right now there are over 800 gynecologists trained to use the colposcope. This means that virtually every hospital associated with a medical school uses the colposcope. And although they are present in many other well-equipped hospitals and a large number of doctor's offices, colposcopes are not available for general use in all hospitals, clinics, and doctor's offices.

If your doctor does not have access to a colposcope, ask about a referral. Otherwise, your doctor can still investigate an abnormal Pap test in other ways. First, your doctor will apply iodine solution (Schiller's test) to your vagina and cervix. This test is capable of identifying abnormal areas requiring biopsy. If your Pap test and/or biopsy reveal dysplasia or worse, cervical conization is necessary — provided that you do not have access to a colposcope or your colposcopy exam is indefinite. While conization has been the time-honored way to investigate women with abnormal Pap tests, colposcopy, when available, is the diagnostic test of choice.

☐ CONIZATION OF THE CERVIX

Conization or cone biopsy — surgical removal of a cone of tissue from the cervix — serves two purposes. As a diagnostic test, gynecologists use it to further investigate certain women with a Pap test suggestive of dysplasia or a more severe condition. (The colposcope has eliminated the need for many diagnostic conizations, however.) Gynecologists also use conization to treat severe dysplasia or very early cancer of the cervix in women who want to have more children. For women with very early cancer who don't want to have more children, hysterectomy is the treatment of choice.

Using general anesthesia, your surgeon removes a cone-shaped segment from the affected area of your cervix. Conization requires several days stay in the hospital. If you develop heavy vaginal bleeding, fever, or abdominal pain after surgery, call your doctor promptly. Otherwise, you can resume sexual activities after your cervix heals in six to eight weeks.

☐ LAPAROTOMY AND LAPAROSCOPY

Until recently, laparotomy was the major way for surgeons to evaluate women with abdominal pain and to carry out tubal ligation. This "look" inside the abdominal and pelvic cavity requires major surgery, several days stay in the hospital, a good deal of expense, and a long recovery period. For this reason, laparotomy is now generally used to establish a diagnosis of cancer of the ovaries and the Fallopian tubes, or remove ovarian cysts when hysterectomy is unnecessary. Because of the deep pelvic location of the ovaries and tubes, nonsurgical diagnostic tests, like the Pap test, are truly impossible. If cancer is found at the time of laparotomy, surgical treatment is usually done at this time.

From time to time, gynecologists use laparotomy to gain access to tie and/or cut the Fallopian tubes for tubal ligation, a method of sterilization. If laparotomy is used for tubal ligation, it is generally done immediately after delivery or other surgery such as abortion or cesarean section. Done at this time, a separate hospital admission becomes unnecessary.

Since the early 1970s, many hospitals have been pioneering a new, much simpler method of achieving nearly the same results of laparotomy at far less expense and physical trauma. A laparoscope (a pencil-like viewing device with a light source) is inserted through a small incision in the navel or lower abdomen. Laparoscopy permits gynecologists to explore the abdominal and pelvic cavity without the major surgery required of laparotomy. Gynecologists commonly use laparoscopy to investigate women with:

> Infertility.
> Endometriosis.
> Pelvic pain or mass.
> Pelvic cancer.
> Diseases of the uterus, ovaries, and Fallopian tubes.
> Pregnancy outside the uterus.
> IUDs that have perforated through the wall of the uterus.

The widest use of laparoscopy is for tubal ligation, a method of sterilization.

Laparoscopy is a brief procedure, taking about 30 minutes. To see the organs clearly, the abdomen is inflated with a harmless gas (carbon dioxide). Through one or two small incisions in the abdomen, the doctor inserts the laparoscope. While laparoscopy is a relatively safe procedure — especially when performed by a doctor well-trained in the technique — there are times when its use is hazardous. If you have any of the following medical conditions, you should not undergo laparoscopy: extreme overweight; hernia; history of extensive pelvic surgery; heart disease; or respiratory disease.

19

CANCER FACTS

Cancer is a frightening word, often associated with "that thing I always dreaded" or "that thing my aunt died of." And, when we discover a cancer symptom such as abnormal bleeding, a lump, wart, or sore that doesn't heal, we often delay going to our doctor. We are afraid that the cancer symptom might be found to be serious. These are normal concerns, especially when you consider that less than 50 years ago, only one in five people were alive five years after cancer treatment. Now, with improved methods of early diagnosis and treatment, the ratio is one in three. This ratio could be even higher if everyone reported all abnormal symptoms to a doctor promptly. Though curing cancer is based on a complex series of events, women whose cancer is diagnosed during the early stages have the best chance for cure. Left untreated, cancer can spread to other parts of the body (metastasize) and eventually cause death.

All women should have regular checkups, with a Pap test. (See Chapter 1, Health Care Checkups.) These checkups help doctors uncover both routine and complex problems. Doctors now know that certain types of cancer *may* be preceded by very early, precancerous conditions. Best of all, most of these conditions are nearly 100 percent curable if treated early. If cancer is diagnosed at an early stage, current treatment allows many women to be cured.

Help yourself and your doctor by taking an active role in your own well-being. Find out your "at risk" status for cancer of the reproductive system and learn the American

Cancer Society's seven warning signals of cancer. The seven warning signs are:

> Change in bowel or bladder habits.
> A sore that does not heal.
> Unusual bleeding or discharge.
> Thickening or lump in the breast or elsewhere.
> Indigestion or difficulty in swallowing.
> Obvious change in wart or mole.
> Nagging cough or hoarseness.

Even though these signals do not always indicate cancer, they may require medical evaluation. If you have any of these symptoms longer than two weeks, see a doctor. Don't wait for your regular checkup or for your symptom to go away by itself.

☐ CANCER AND ITS CAUSES

Clinicians, laboratory scientists, and epidemiologists have all tried to understand the nature and cause of cancer — a colony of very abnormal, runaway cells that multiply rapidly and without purpose. Arising from one cell that has the ability to reproduce, cancer cells can invade healthy tissue and spread to other parts of the body. Cancer can also occur at any age in any part of the body. According to current statistics from the National Cancer Institute, about 12 percent of all women develop cancer sometime in their lives. Of these women, 26 percent develop cancer of the breast; reproductive system (21 percent); colon-rectum (15 percent); other digestive organs (9 percent); leukemia and lymphoma (7 percent); urinary tract (4 percent); and all other (18 percent).

It isn't always known why a normal cell turns into a cancer cell and then reproduces into a colony of cancer cells. Certain viruses, heredity, environmental agents, and a combination of these factors have already been implicated in the development of various types of cancer. For example, tobacco is responsible for more cancer cases (lung, bladder, and mouth) than any other known agent. Additionally, exposure to certain estrogens, radiation, sunlight, and occupational products such as chemicals and asbestos have also been identified as cancer-causing (carcinogenic) agents. Most of these cancers can be prevented by avoiding or reducing contact with these agents. This is because the risk of developing cancer is often related to the amount and length of exposure to these carcinogenic agents. Unfortunately, many other, less well-understood cancers do not have such practical measures. But right now, researchers are trying to understand the nature of certain viruses and heredity in addition to identifying other carcinogenic agents to help prevent more cancers.

□ CANCER OF THE REPRODUCTIVE SYSTEM

Cervical Cancer

Over the past 25 years, researchers have collected a great deal of new information about the nature of cervical conditions. It is now known that cervical cancer *may* be preceded by early cervical conditions which usually don't cause symptoms. In fact, cervical cells may go through a series of changes. They may change from normal to abnormal (dysplasia or abnormal cells covering the cervix); to very early cancer (also known as cancer *in situ* which only involves the top layer of the cervix); to invasive cancer which invades the deeper layers of the cervix.

A test now exists—and has existed for nearly 30 years in doctors' offices and clinics—that helps detect cervical conditions. It's called the Pap test or Pap smear—a simple, painless, quick laboratory test for detection of abnormal cells from the cervix. Best of all, the Pap test makes it possible to discover dysplasia and very early cancer—symptom-free conditions which are almost 100 percent curable if treated early. It actually turns out that if all women had a Pap test as part of their regular checkup, most invasive cancer of the cervix could be prevented. But cancer of the cervix — including very early cancer — is currently the second most common cancer in women. Right now invasive cancer still accounts for six percent of all cancer in women and 30 percent of all cancer of the reproductive system.

"At Risk" Women. Some women run a greater chance of having cervical changes than other women. These women are considered to be "at risk." Though the exact cause is uncertain, sexual intercourse is somehow involved in the development of these conditions. Having sexual intercourse in one's teens or having numerous male partners are two risk factors which increase the chance of developing a cervical condition. These conditions are also more common in women who don't have access to regular medical checkups. Also, researchers have suggested that women with a history of herpes virus type 2 may be "at risk." Herpes virus type 2 is a sexually-transmitted infection characterized by small, painful blisters on the genitals. (See Chapter 4, Genital Herpes.)

All of these conditions tend to develop at different times in a woman's life. One of these conditions, dysplasia, usually develops in 25- to 35-year-old women and may even develop in women in their late teens and early twenties. Though very early cancer usually develops in women who are between the ages of 30 and 40, it is being diagnosed more frequently in women in their twenties. Invasive cancer is primarily a condition of premenopausal women who are 40 to 50 years of age.

Symptoms. Dysplasia and very early cancer usually don't cause symptoms. Invasive cancer generally causes abnormal vaginal bleeding (especially after intercourse), spotting between menstrual periods, after douching, or bleeding after the menopause.

Diagnosis. The Pap test is the best way to *screen* all women for dysplasia, very early cancer, and invasive cancer. If your

Pap test suggests dysplasia or if a more severe condition is present, it doesn't always mean that you have a precancerous or cancerous condition. It does, however, mean that you need to have other diagnostic tests to find out why the Pap test is abnormal before your doctor starts any type of treatment.

Tests which your doctor can perform in the office, with little discomfort, include the application of iodine solution (Schiller's test) to your cervix. If certain areas on your cervix appear abnormal during the exam, your doctor may remove a tiny amount of tissue (biopsy) for microscopic examination and diagnosis.

A colposcope — a diagnostic instrument that simply magnifies the surface of the vagina and cervix — may be used for the exam. (See Chapter 18.) The colposcope helps gynecologists pinpoint suspicious areas for biopsy. Although the colposcope is helpful, it is not required and is not always available. If your doctor or clinic does not have access to a colposcope (ask about a referral), your doctor can still investigate an abormal Pap test by using iodine solution for biopsy. Additionally, your doctor may take tissue scrapings of your cervical canal. Brief hospitalization may also be necessary for D and C and conization. (See Chapter 18.)

Treatment. Treatment varies among medical centers and from woman to woman. How dysplasia is treated depends on its severity. For women with mild dysplasia, treatment may not be necessary. When treatment is necessary, your doctor can usually do it in the office with little discomfort. In many women, treatment involves cryosurgery, where abnormal areas on the cervix are frozen and destroyed by a probe. In some women, treatment involves hot cauterization, where abnormal areas on the cervix are burned and destroyed by an electrical probe. For some women, brief hospitalization may be necessary for conization, where abnormal tissue is surgically removed from the cervix and cervical canal.

Treatment for very early cancer may involve conization, cryosurgery, or hot cauterization. Occasionally, further treatment may be necessary. Hysterectomy is the treatment of choice, however, for women who don't want to have any more children. (See Chapter 18.) All women should schedule regular checkups after any type of treatment for very early cancer.

Treatment for invasive cancer depends upon the extent of cancer discovered at the diagnostic exam. Treatment may require surgery, radiation therapy, or a combination of the two. Surgery involves radical hysterectomy. Radiation therapy, which destroys cancer cells and some surrounding normal cells, may also be used. The length of radiation therapy varies. Typically, a combination of internal and external radiation therapy is used. In internal radiation — requiring brief hospitalization — radioactive material such as radium is inserted into the uterus and vagina. In external radiation therapy — usually given on an outpatient basis — a machine delivers radiation to the affected area. Treatment for invasive cancer may also require chemotherapy.

Endometrial Cancer

Cancer of the endometrium (lining of the uterus) is the second most common cancer of the reproductive system. On the increase for the past 15 years, it currently accounts for seven percent of all cancer in women and 36 percent of all cancer of the reproductive system. While cancer of the breast and cervix are currently the most common types of cancer in women — if rates continue to increase — endometrial cancer may challenge their position in the next ten years. Researchers have offered numerous explanations for the dramatic rise including improved cancer reporting plus more accurate methods of cancer diagnosis. But, since the mid-1970s, several studies have associated the rise with increased use of estrogen replacement therapy during the menopause. And this last explanation — according to statisticians — may be partly responsible for the rising number of endometrial cancers. (More about that later.)

Like cervical cancer, endometrial cancer *may* be preceded by early precancerous conditions which are usually 100 percent curable if treated early. It is now known that endometrial cells may change from normal to abnormal (certain types of precancerous hyperplasia or abnormal cells covering the endometium); to very early cancer (also called cancer *in situ* which only involves the top layer of the endometrium); to invasive cancer which invades the deeper layers of the endometrium.

"At Risk" Women. Women who run a greater chance of developing endometrial conditions than other women currently include those with one or more of the following risk factors: over age 50; abnormal vaginal bleeding; late menopause (after age 50); overweight, high blood pressure, diabetes; or infertility.

Since 1975, several different groups of researchers have reported that women who take estrogen replacement therapy during the menopause are anywhere from four to fifteen times more likely to develop endometrial cancer than women who don't. (See Chapter 21, Estrogen Replacement Therapy.)

Symptoms. Abnormal vaginal bleeding is the most common symptom. Generally this starts off as light spotting and discharge. Over time, bleeding becomes heavier and more frequent.

Diagnosis. Definite diagnosis requires tissue scrapings of the cervical canal and lining of the uterus (D and C) for microscopic examination.

Although the Pap test is occasionally helpful, it is not a very reliable screening test for this type of cancer. For this reason, more and more doctors now use endometrial aspiration. In this diagnostic test — a screening test for women at "high-risk" for endometrial cancer — cells from the uterus are safely and painlessly removed for laboratory study.

Treatment. For women with certain types of precancerous hyperplasia and very early cancer, hysterectomy is usually the treatment of choice. Treatment of invasive cancer depends upon the extent of cancer found at the diagnostic exam. It usually involves hysterectomy with removal of both ovaries and Fallopian tubes. This may be combined with radiation therapy.

Ovarian Cancer

Ranking as the third most common cancer of the reproductive system, ovarian cancer accounts for five percent of all cancer in women and 25 percent of all cancer of the reproductive system. But the worst aspect of ovarian cancer is that its yearly death rate exceeds that of endometrial and cervical cancer combined.

"At Risk" Women. Women who run a greater chance of developing ovarian cancer than other women currently include those with one or more of the following risk factors: over age 45; heavy menstrual bleeding before the menopause; infertility; or a history of ovarian cancer among close relatives.

Symptoms. Ovarian cancer is very difficult to detect at an early stage. This is because the ovaries are located deep in the pelvic cavity, making early detection very difficult. Abnormal vaginal bleeding is not usually a symptom, as it is with other cancers. Abdominal discomfort, swelling, and indigestion may be present, creating the sensation of middle-age indigestion, rather than an underlying cancer.

Diagnosis. Only surgical exploration of the pelvic cavity (laparotomy) for a suspicious ovarian mass provides a definite diagnosis. (See Chapter 18). If cancer is present, surgical treatment is usually done at this time.

Treatment. Treatment depends upon the extent of cancer found at the diagnostic exam. It usually involves hysterectomy with removal of both ovaries and Fallopian tubes. Radiation therapy and chemotherapy may also be used.

Vulvar Cancer

Cancer of the vulva is a relatively uncommon condition. Women who run a greater chance of developing vulvar cancer than other women currently include those with one or more of the following risk factors: aged 60 to 70; overweight; or high blood pressure.

Symptoms. While vulvar cancer may start off causing intense itching, redness, and soreness of the vulva, the most common symptom is a lump or painful ulcer.

Diagnosis. Definite diagnosis requires removal of a tiny amount of tissue from abnormal areas (biopsy) for microscopic examination.

Treatment. Treatment usually involves surgical removal of the vulva and underlying tissue (radical vulvectomy) plus removal of the surrounding lymph nodes. Radiation therapy may also be used.

Vaginal Cancer

Cancer of the vagina is an uncommon condition of the postmenopausal years. So far, researchers have not been able to identify any risk factors for postmenopausal women. Yet, in 1971, a group of researchers reported an association between a very rare cancer of the vagina and daughters exposed *in utero* to stilbestrol. Until then, this type of cancer was virtually unknown in women under age 50. (See Chapter 16.)

Symptoms. Common symptoms include abnormal vaginal bleeding or discharge, especially after intercourse or douching.

Diagnosis. Diagnosis requires iodine solution (Schiller's test) followed by removal of a tiny amount of tissue from abnormal areas (biopsy) for microscopic examination. Though the Pap test is helpful, it is not always reliable for detecting this type of cancer.

Treatment. While treatment varies from woman to woman, it often involves radical hysterectomy. When it is necessary to remove the vagina, an artificial one can be constructed to replace it, making sexual intercourse possible after the vagina has healed. Radiation therapy may also be used.

Fallopian Tube Cancer

Cancer of the Fallopian tube is the least common cancer of the reproductive system, primarily affecting women between the ages of 45 and 60. Women "at risk" for developing this type of cancer have a history of infertility.

Symptoms. Common symptoms include cramp-like abdominal pain and honey-colored vaginal discharge. Abnormal vaginal bleeding and abdominal swelling may also be present.

Diagnosis. As with ovarian cancer, only surgical exploration of the pelvic cavity (laparotomy) for a suspicious mass provides a definite diagnosis. If cancer is present, surgical treatment is usually done at this time.

Treatment. Treatment usually involves hysterectomy with removal of both ovaries and Fallopian tubes. Chemotherapy and/or hormone therapy may also be used.

☐ TREATMENT AND SIDE EFFECTS

From the time of cancer diagnosis through treatment, you have the right to be well-informed by your doctor. (See Chapter 1, Patient Rights.) Before treatment, your doctor should discuss various issues with you, your family, and/or one of your close friends. Your doctor should explain the reasons for recommending the chosen treatment in relation to the extent of your cancer. In addition, you and your doctor should discuss the risks, side effects, and benefits of treatment in addition to any alternative treatment that exists for you. As a patient, you have the right to complete and current information concerning your diagnosis, treatment, and prognosis. Make sure you understand what your doctor is saying. If you don't, say so.

Side effects from cancer treatment vary from woman to woman.

Surgery. Complete recovery from hysterectomy usually takes several months. See Chapter 18 for common side effects following hysterectomy. If you develop any of these problems, be sure to contact your doctor promptly.

Radiation Therapy. The length of radiation therapy varies. External radiation therapy is usually given on an outpatient basis for several weeks, while internal radiation therapy requires brief hospitalization. Radiation therapy has greatly improved over the past ten years or so. The side effects that used to be so common are now very rare. At this point, minor skin reactions, nausea, vomiting, and a feeling of tiredness may be side effects of external radiation. Radioactive material inserted into the uterus or vagina may cause redness, warmth, swelling, and sometimes pain. The walls of the vagina may tighten and stick together after internal or external radiation. Periodic sexual intercourse or manual dilation of the vagina with a plexiglas mold can minimize this problem, however. A mold, along with proper instructions, is available from your doctor.

Be sure to keep your radiotherapist aware of any problems. It is possible to have your treatment plan modified or medications prescribed to ease any uncomfortable side effects.

Chemotherapy. Most chemotherapy is given in the doctor's office or hospital outpatient department. In some cases, short periods of hospitalization may be necessary. Chemotherapy is known to cause certain side effects. Common problems may include: nausea and vomiting; diarrhea; mouth sores; and temporary hair loss. Be sure to keep your chemotherapist aware of any problems. It is possible to have your treatment plan modified or medications prescribed to ease any uncomfortable side effects.

Regular checkups are a must for women with a history of cancer. After treatment, ask your doctor how often to schedule your checkups. Of course, if you develop any abnormal symptoms between visits, call your doctor promptly. Generally, these checkups include thorough gynecologic physical exams, Pap tests, and other laboratory tests. These checkups are essential, so be sure to keep your appointments. These exams enable doctors to provide treatment at the earliest possible time for any condition requiring further treatment.

☐ PROVEN AND UNPROVEN METHODS OF CANCER TREATMENT

Cancer of the reproductive system requires treatment by an experienced doctor. (See Chapter 18.) The important thing is to receive the best care you possible can. This means that you should be treated by a gynecologist experienced in the treatment of cancer, rather than by a doctor who treats an occasional case of cancer. (Incidentally, since the early 1970s, a new subspecialty of gynecology, called gynecologic oncology, enables gynecologists to receive specialty training in gynecologic cancer surgery. At this time, there are not that many of these doctors around.) If your doctor tells you "nothing can be done," get a second medical opinion. Don't spend a lot of time shopping around for a doctor who will tell you what you want to hear—that you really don't have cancer or that surgery, for example, is unnecessary.

Your own gynecologist may be able to give you the best treatment. If your doctor is not experienced in treating cancer, you should be referred to a doctor who is. Or, if you prefer, you can contact your local American Cancer Society for advice. While the American Cancer Society does not have a policy of making referrals to specific doctors, your local office can give you general advice about what to do and how to locate your own doctor. In addition, the National Cancer Institute has established an Office of Cancer Communications. This office provides public information and helps cancer patients and their doctors find names and addresses of cancer specialists nearest home. (See Readings and Resources.)

Because the treatment of cancer is complex, hospital-based specialists trained in surgery, radiotherapy, and chemotherapy generally work together as a team. This medical team, coupled with the support of nurses, social workers, clergy, psychiatrists, and other professionals, is necessary for proper cancer care. In contrast to this organized medical team, various organizations, peddlers, and mail order companies solicit fraudulent cancer "cures." Although these cures are not of any proven benefit (and may even be dangerous), women spend thousands of dollars yearly in search of the perfect cancer cure. Consumers interested in health have used caustic salves, health diets, pills, vaccines, and so forth. Not only are these cures useless and even dangerous, but women using them usually delay needed medical attention when early diagnosis and treatment can help in curing cancer. If you ever have doubts about any type of cancer treatment you are considering or have ever received, check it out with the American Cancer Society. This organization keeps an up-to-date list of unproven methods of cancer treatment.

Right now, treatments of proven benefit include surgery, radiation therapy, and chemotherapy. Cancer treatment varies from woman to woman. What is good for one woman may not be advisable in another. Only a doctor — not schemes promoted by the health-quackery field — can reach a decision about proper cancer management.

☐ EXPERIMENTAL CANCER TREATMENT

Both clinicians and laboratory scientists agree that experimental studies with humans are necessary for progress toward the most effective cancer treatment. But, at the same time, lawyers, sociologists, economists, theologians, and doctors have argued that experimental studies may present severe legal, social, and ethical problems. While many experimental studies continue to make valuable contributions toward the treatment of cancer, an obvious dilemma exists. Final decision regarding participation in an experimental study rests with the cancer patient. If you ever consider participating in an experimental study, be sure to thoroughly discuss the risks and benefits of treatment with your doctor.

Most experimental studies are conducted with limited groups of patients selected by the medical researcher in charge of the study. These studies are generally conducted in institutions affiliated with a medical school, the National Cancer Institute (a division of the National Institutes of Health), or private cancer institutes. If you agree to participate in a study sponsored by one of these institutions, don't worry about being a guinea pig. All of these studies must undergo very careful scientific and ethical review before any cancer patient can receive treatment. Moreover, as a patient, you will receive — at the least — the best available treatment for your cancer. At the most, you may receive a new therapy that may even be more effective.

Since the early 1970s, federal and state governments have legally required that all patients must be provided with an explanation of the treatment plan; its risks, side effects, and benefits; an explanation of any alternative treatment that would be advantageous; and indications that the patient may withdraw from the study at any time. This explanation, termed "informed consent," may be verbal but is usually written. (Both forms are legally valid.) Discussion of informed consent should take place *before* the experimental study begins. Any study lacking informed consent is truly unethical. Fortunately, many professional organizations have adopted codes of ethics to guide human experimentation, making unethical studies events of the past.

Experimental clinical studies generally investigate the value of a new therapy (for example, postoperative chemotherapy for breast cancer) or the merits of existing therapies which are in dispute (for example, radical mastectomy versus less radical surgery for breast cancer). The goal of any experimental study is to evaluate which (if any) of two or more types of cancer treatment is most effective.

To enable the medical researcher to identify the better treatment, patients are assigned into a treatment or a non-treatment group. The treatment or study group receives the drug or other therapeutic procedure under investigation. The nontreatment or control group, for example, either receives a different treatment or the same treatment as the study group but at a different dose. The assignment of a patient to a study or control group is usually random. This means that group assignment is beyond the control of the researcher and patient. Only chance determines who gets into one group or another. Researchers commonly use randomization because it is considered to be the best way to conduct an experimental study. A few researchers disagree with randomization. Instead, the researcher and, at times, the patient may choose the group assignment. Although this latter type of study is rare and presents greater statistical problems for the researcher, it is more considerate of the cancer patient. It may even obtain better results for the patient. In addition to random group assignment, in some studies both the patient and researcher do not know to which group the patient has been assigned (double-blind).

Depending upon the treatment under investigation, the length of an experimental study may range from several weeks to several years. During and after the completion of the study, you are expected to schedule checkup exams at regular intervals throughout the year. Generally, these checkups include thorough gynecologic physical exams, Pap tests, and other laboratory tests to evaluate your response to treatment. These checkups are essential, so be sure to keep your appointments. If you develop any kind of symptom or side effect between visits, call your doctor promptly. It may be necessary for you to stop treatment or have your treatment plan modified.

20

BREAST CANCER

Not so long ago, no one talked much about breast cancer — the most common type of cancer in women. Since the early 1970s — especially after Betty Ford and Happy Rockefeller underwent surgery for breast cancer — many women are now talking frankly about their experiences. Not only that, but both the medical journals and the media have frequent accounts about "The 'At Risk' Groups," "Radical Versus Less Radical Surgery," and "The Latest Advances in Chemotherapy." Indeed, women have come into their doctors' offices waving articles from this or that magazine or newspaper demanding answers to all their questions. But right now your doctor cannot give answers to all your questions. This is because medical authorities — around the world — disagree on many points.

Over the years, there have been many advances in both the diagnosis and treatment of breast cancer. Even so, here are the disturbing facts. According to 1979 figures from the American Cancer Society, breast cancer now strikes 106,000 American women every year. One out of 14 women (or 7 percent) is destined to get breast cancer during her lifetime. Every woman over age 35 is "at risk," especially those over age 50. Moreover, breast cancer causes more deaths than any other type of cancer — an estimated 34,200 a year. By the time of diagnosis, cancer has spread outside the breast in 40 percent of all women. From these figures, it is obvious that breast cancer is a potential threat to many women.

Help yourself and your doctor by taking an active role in

your own well-being. Find out your "at risk" status, examine your breasts every month, and see a doctor for regular check-ups. If you discover a breast lump, see a doctor promptly. Don't wait to see if your breast lump gets bigger or causes pain, since early breast cancers are usually small and painless.

As will be seen in this chapter, early diagnosis and treatment offer the best chance for cure.

☐ **"AT RISK" WOMEN**

Who is most likely to develop breast cancer? Currently, there is no way of pinpointing *the* woman destined to develop it. Even so, breast cancer does seem more common among certain women as compared to others. Women over age 50 and those between the ages of 35 and 50 who meet one or more of the following criteria are considered to be "at risk." Though "at risk" women are more likely to develop breast cancer than other women, all women are susceptible.

Regardless of whether you are "at risk" or not, be sure to examine your breasts every month. If — according to your doctor — you are at *high* rather than *low*-risk for developing breast cancer, your doctor may recommend a yearly mammographic screening exam.

Risk Factors

Risk factors in their general order of importance are:

History of Cancer. About seven to ten percent of women with a history of cancer in one breast develop cancer in the opposite breast. Additionally, women with a history of cancer of the endometrium (lining of the uterus) or ovary are at higher risk of developing breast cancer than other women.

Age. Under age 35, the risk is minimal. All women over age 35 are "at risk." Risk increases with age and about 75 percent of all breast cancer occurs in women over age 50.

Breast cancer is almost unknown before puberty and is very rare in women under age 20.

Family History. Women with a history of breast cancer in the immediate family (mother or sister) have two to three times the risk of developing breast cancer than other women. Breast cancer tends to develop about ten years earlier in this group of "at risk" women. Also, women whose mothers had breast cancer in both breasts before menopause are at especially high-risk.

Late Menopause. Women with a late menopause (55 years of age or older) are at higher risk than those with early menopause (before 45 years of age). Late menopause implies that a woman probably has menstruated for more than 35 years.

Age at Birth of First Child. Women who have never delivered a baby or who delivered their first baby after age 30 are at higher risk than women who delivered before age 30.

Age at First Menstrual Period. Women who began to menstruate early (before age 11) are at higher risk than those who began to menstruate late (over 15 years).

Benign Breast Disease. Women with certain types of fibrocystic disease appear to develop breast cancer about two to three times more often than other women.

This profile is at best a general guide. If you fulfill all of the criteria, you are not destined to develop breast cancer. By the same token, if you do not fulfill any of these risk factors, you are not immune. Any woman can develop breast cancer.

☐ **SYMPTOMS**

About 95 percent of all women with a breast lump discover it by self-examination. Most breast lumps are not cancer. In fact, about eight out of ten breast lumps requiring biopsy are not cancer, but one of the benign breast diseases such as fibrocystic disease or fibroadenoma.

If you discover any of the following symptoms, arrange an appointment promptly with the doctor or clinic you regularly use:

Breast lump.
Breast pain and/or tenderness.
Nipple discharge.
Dimpling or puckering of breast skin.
Any unusual skin or nipple changes.

□ **DIAGNOSIS**

Your doctor will thoroughly examine your breasts and decide if the breast symptom requires further investigation. If it does, your doctor will then refer you to a surgeon who will very thoroughly examine your breasts. (More about that later.) If the breast lump feels suspicious, your surgeon will arrange one or more of the following screening tests such as mammography, xeroradiography, or thermography. Biopsy is necessary if any screening test reveals a suspicious-looking or positive breast lump. Doctors use the results from all of these diagnostic tests — but most importantly biopsy — to determine if the breast lump is likely to be breast cancer or one of the benign breast diseases.

Mammography

Mammography, or low-dose X-ray of the breast, is currently the most accurate nonsurgical diagnostic test. It is capable of detecting benign breast disease, suspicious-looking areas, and definite breast cancer.

Though mammography can detect breast cancer before the lump is too small to be felt, it has become the subject of controversy. In 1971 — in cooperation with the American Cancer Society — the National Cancer Institute established 27 Breast

Cancer Detection Demonstration Projects across the country. Right now these projects are screening nearly 300,000 women a year for breast cancer. From 1972 to August 1976, these two groups advocated routine mammographic screening for all women over age 35. In August 1976, however, they revised their guidelines to include only "at risk" women between the ages of 35 and 50 and all women over age 50. They revised their guidelines because numerous medical authorities argued that the cancer-inducing potential of X-ray mammography may actually outweigh the benefits of early detection. Meanwhile, if you agree to participate in routine mammographic screening, be sure to ask your doctor about both its risks and benefits.

Xeroradiography

Xeroradiography is another type of X-ray exam that produces a picture of the breast on a Xerox plate instead of X-ray film. (Low-dose mammography and xeroradiography use about the same amount of radiation as a complete dental X-ray exam but more than a chest X-ray.)

Thermography

By scanning the breast with an infrared camera, thermography charts heat patterns of the breast with a Polaroid camera. Cancer of the breast is usually hotter than normal breast tissue. But benign conditions can also show "hot spots" or false-positive readings. Thermography is a safe and inexpensive test that is being used along with mammography and xeroradiography. At present, this is the only method that does not use radiation. Unfortunately, it is the least available and the least accurate of all the methods.

Biopsy

This is the *only* way to determine if the breast lump is cancer or benign breast disease. This is because a definite diagnosis depends on microscopic examination of the breast biopsy by a pathologist.

Right now there are several tests that can be done in the office or clinic, usually without anesthesia. Your doctor may first do a *needle aspiration* (fluid removal of cells) to see if it is a cyst. If the lump remains and does not collapse, surgical biopsy is necessary. Surgical biopsy is also necessary if mammography reveals any suspicious areas or if a fibrocystic lump persists or flares up one to two months after needle aspiration.

Surgical biopsy, usually done under general anesthesia, may be either incisional (partial removal of the lump) or excisional (total removal of the lump). Most surgeons prefer excisional biopsy for its thoroughness. This is because inaccurate diagnoses are possible when only part of the lump is removed for microscopic diagnosis.

If the breast lump is cancer and mastectomy is the treatment of choice, you have two options which you may wish to discuss with your surgeon before surgery:

• Have your biopsy done as a separate operative procedure before mastectomy. This means that you could discuss alternatives with your doctor, your family, and/or one of your close friends before further surgery. By doing this, you avoid unexpected mastectomy under the same anesthesia. If you choose this option, mastectomy is usually done shortly after biospy. (A brief delay is not hazardous to cure.)

• Have your biopsy and mastectomy done at the same time. Many women choose this option. They prefer to have the entire procedure of biopsy and mastectomy undertaken with one anesthesia, without discussion.

Other

Most surgeons routinely perform certain diagnostic tests before surgery. These tests are necessary since breast cancer — like any type of cancer — can spread to other parts of the body such as to the bones, liver, and lungs. For this reason, surgeons often use a chest X-ray, bone scan, possibly a liver scan, and various blood tests to measure the extent of cancer. The findings of all these tests assist your doctor in choosing the best treatment for you.

☐ COMMON BENIGN BREAST DISEASES

If the breast lump is not cancer, it is one of the benign breast diseases that affect many women in their menstruating years.

Fibrocystic disease is the most common type of breast lump. While it does not appear to be precancerous, women with certain types of fibrocystic disease develop breast cancer two to three times more often than other women. It usually makes its appearance during the thirties and is very common in the forties. Unlike breast cancer, which continues to increase with advancing age, fibrocystic disease is rare after the menopause. With one exception, it may reappear in menopausal women using estrogen replacement therapy.

Fibrocystic disease can appear in a variety of forms: both breasts may be only painful and tender; breasts may feel fuller, heavier, and a bit lumpy; or, one or more cysts — small or large — may be felt. Women with fibrocystic disease often notice breast changes throughout their menstrual cycle. Generally, symptoms are worse before the menstrual period and then subside or disappear after the period. Likewise, cysts may come and go with the period, remain stable, or disappear completely from time to time.

If you have these symptoms, you may have fibrocystic disease, though only a doctor can tell for sure. If you have fibrocystic disease, you can help yourself and your doctor if you practice monthly breast self-examination. While examining your breasts, pay attention to the changes that occur in your breasts with each menstrual cycle. Only by becoming familiar with your breasts under normal conditions will you recognize something different that a doctor should check.

Fibroadenoma is the third most common type of breast

lump, exceeded only by fibrocystic disease and breast cancer. Fibroadenomas can occur in teenagers but are more common in women in their twenties and thirties. Fibroadenomas can range in size from small peas to grapes. Unlike fibrocystic disease, they don't usually cause pain or tenderness.

If you discover any type of lump in your breasts, see a doctor promptly. Though eight out of ten breast lumps requiring biopsy are benign breast disease, only a doctor can tell for sure by careful breast examination and diagnostic tests.

☐ TREATMENT

Most breast cancer is treated by general surgeons and less frequently by gynecologists. The important thing is to receive the best care you possibly can. This means that you should be treated by a doctor experienced in the treatment of breast cancer, rather than by a doctor who treats an occasional case of breast cancer. And, if your doctor tells you "nothing can be done," get a second medical opinion. Don't spend a lot of time shopping around for a doctor who will tell you what you want to hear, though — that you really don't have cancer or that surgery, for example, is unnecessary.

Your own doctor may be able to give you the best treatment. If your doctor is not experienced in this area, you should be referred to a doctor who is. Or, if you prefer, you can contact your local American Cancer Society for advice. While the American Cancer Society does not have a policy of making referrals to specific doctors, your local office can give you general advice about what to do and how to locate your own physician. In addition, the National Cancer Institute has established an Office of Cancer Communications. This office provides public information and helps cancer patients and their doctors find names and addresses of cancer specialists nearest home. (See Readings and Resources.)

From the time of cancer diagnosis through treatment, you have the right to be well-informed by your doctor. (See

Chapter 1, Patient Rights.) Before treatment, your doctor should discuss various issues with you, your family, and/or one of your close friends. Your doctor should explain the reasons for recommending the chosen treatment in relation to the extent of your breast cancer. In addition, you and your doctor should discuss the risks, side effects, and benefits of treatment in addition to any alternative treatment that exists for you. As a patient, you have the right to complete and current information concerning your diagnosis, treatment, and prognosis. Make sure you understand what your doctor is saying. If you don't, say so.

Whether the cancer is confined to the breast, has spread to the lymph nodes, or to other parts of the body, is a measure of the cancer "stage," or how far the cancer has spread. (See Table 13.) Before treatment, all breast cancers are staged by evaluating the findings from the various diagnostic tests. After staging and consultation with several physicians, your doctor recommends a treatment plan that may involve surgery, radiation therapy, chemotherapy, or a combination of the three. Surgery is the most widely used form of treatment. Treatment, however, varies from woman to woman. Numerous variables such as size and location of the breast

---

TABLE 13. Breast Cancer Stage

STAGE	EXTENT OF BREAST CANCER
Stage I	Breast lump is small (less than 3/4 inch), may be attached to breast muscles, and all lymph nodes are cancer-free.
Stage II	Breast lump is no more than 2 inches and may be attached to breast muscles. Some lymph nodes may be involved with cancer.
Stage III	Breast lump is large (bigger than 2 inches) and is usually attached to breast muscles, chest wall, or skin. Lymph nodes are often involved with cancer.
Stage IV	Breast cancer has spread to other parts of the body.

lump, extent of breast cancer, cell type, and so forth influence treatment choice. Treatment that is best for one woman may not be advisable in another. The ultimate goal of any treatment plan is cure: elimination of all the cancer.

Surgery

Numerous surgical procedures are currently being used to treat operable breast cancer: lumpectomy; simple or total mastectomy; modified radical mastectomy; and radical mastectomy. Right now, there is a lot of controversy around which of these procedures will remove *all* of the cancer and cure the greatest number of women. Retrospective studies have tried — by reviewing medical records of treated cases of breast cancer — to compare the prognosis of women treated with each of the above procedures. Due to poor study design and faulty statistical analysis, there are many defects in these research studies. This has made comparison between studies very difficult, if not impossible.

At present, the most statistically valid and popular way to evaluate treatment effect is the randomized clinical study. (See Chapter 19, Experimental Cancer Treatment.) In this, patients are randomly selected for one of several methods of treatment. Many ongoing clinical studies are trying to determine, for example, if less radical surgery (used alone or with radiation therapy) can work just as well — in certain groups of women — as radical surgery. Until all the results are in (at least ten years of follow-up after treatment are necessary before there can be any strong hope for cure), the modified and radical mastectomy remain the standard method of treating operable breast cancer. What evidence there is strongly suggests that in the long run, radical rather than less radical surgery may save many more lives. In any case, there will never be one best treatment for all women.

Methods have varied over the years between lesser and more extensive surgery. (See Table 14.) The Halsted radical mastectomy, developed by Dr. William Halsted in the 1880s, is currently the most widely used method in most medical centers throughout the world, because many surgeons feel it

TABLE 14. Breast Surgery

TYPE OF SURGERY	WHAT GETS REMOVED			
	Lump	Breast	Surrounding Lymph Nodes	Pectoral Muscles
Lumpectomy	*			
Simple or total mastectomy	*	*		
Modified radical mastectomy	*	*	*	
Radical mastectomy	*	*	*	*

* Indicates removal

is the only way to remove all the tumor. At the other end of the spectrum is excision of the tumor (lumpectomy), which has received a lot of attention lately. Unfortunately, the proponents of lumpectomy place a lot of reliance on unproven theory and disregard well-documented facts concerning the nature of breast cancer. Also, their data, which they use to support their arguments, does not hold up after careful scientific review. It lumpectomy were as effective as mastectomy, it would be used more frequently. Since many breast cancers are "multicentric" (occur throughout the breast), simply removing the breast lump may not remove *all* of the tumor.

Between the extremes of lumpectomy and radical mastectomy are simple or total mastectomy and the modified radical mastectomy. More and more surgeons are switching from the radical to the modified radical mastectomy as their routine breast cancer operation. One of the advantages of the modified is cosmetic. Unlike the radical mastectomy, it doesn't remove the pectoral muscles on the chest wall which are responsible for shoulder and arm strength. (With proper exercises, however, other muscles can be trained to do the job.) Also, with the pectoral muscles in place, the chest doesn't have such a hollow-looking appearance.

Side effects from surgery vary from woman to woman. Generally, a lumpectomy will cause little discomfort, while a modified or radical mastectomy will cause discomfort for several weeks following surgery. Common side effects after these mastectomies include: arm weakness immediately following surgery and arm swelling (edema) a few weeks or months after surgery. Arm weakness is caused by loss of certain muscles and ligaments. A few days after surgery, a nurse or physical therapist, under your surgeon's supervision, exercises your arm and encourages you to do these exercises both in the hospital and at home. Edema is caused by removal of the lymph nodes and channels — formerly responsible for draining fluid from the breast area and arm. Proper exercises and gentle massage help to relieve the swelling. Later, new lymph channels develop and the swelling generally subsides.

Radiation Therapy

Radiation therapy, which destroys cancer cells and some surrounding normal cells, may be used. In external radiation therapy — usually given on an outpatient basis for about five to six weeks — a machine delivers radiation to the affected breast. Often radiation is used with other types of treatment. For example, it is sometimes given before surgery to reduce the size of the tumor or after surgery when cancerous lymph nodes are discovered. Depending on tumor characteristics, it may supplement a less radical type of surgery. In some cases, it may even be the only type of treatment.

Radiation therapy has greatly improved over the past ten years or so. The side effects that used to be fairly common — swollen arms and burned skin — are now very rare. At this point, minor skin reactions, nausea, vomiting, and a feeling of tiredness may be side effects of radiation. Be sure to keep your radiotherapist aware of any problems. It is possible to have your treatment plan modified or medications prescribed to ease any uncomfortable side effects.

Chemotherapy

A drug or drugs taken orally or by injection, chemotherapy also works by destroying cancer cells. A chemotherapeutic treatment plan may involve one drug or a combination of several chemotherapeutic agents. Most chemotherapy is given in the doctor's office or hospital outpatient department. In some cases, short periods of hospitalization may be necessary.

Until recently, chemotherapy was used to relieve symptoms but was not curative. Chemotherapy after surgery, when cancerous lymph nodes are discovered, is currently being investigated on a cooperative basis among many hospitals. So far, preliminary results show an improved cure rate for premenopausal women. Long-term follow-up of these women is in progress to determine its effectiveness. This form of treatment, however, may prove to be a significant contribution to the management of breast cancer.

Chemotherapy is known to cause certain side effects. Common problems may include: nausea and vomiting; diarrhea; mouth sores; and temporary hair loss. Be sure to keep your chemotherapist aware of any difficulties. It is possible to have your treatment plan modified or medications prescribed to ease any uncomfortable side effects.

Other

Radiation therapy and/or chemotherapy are often used to treat advanced cancer (extending outside the breast) and recurrent cancer (disease appearing after recovery). Moreover, hormone treatment — in the form of surgery or drugs — may also be used to treat certain women. The aim of this method is to actually change each woman's hormonal environment. This means that in menstruating women — who are still producing estrogens — the ovaries and/or adrenal glands may be surgically removed. In postmenopausal women — who are not producing estrogens — estrogen replacement therapy may be prescribed.

Some well-equipped hospitals are now pioneering a new test, the estrogen receptor test. Whether or not to use hormone therapy is based on the results of tissue taken at the time of surgery. It seems that women with a positive test may respond better to hormone therapy than women with a negative test.

☐ AFTER MASTECTOMY

Emotional Reactions

A wide variety of attitudes toward mastectomy exist. Contrary to what some people say, mastectomy should not change you as a person. Of all the women who have had mastectomies, many have adjusted quickly and gone on to live busy, active lives. This is because mastectomy does not make you less of a woman, put an end to your social or sex life, or make you less attractive or desirable — even though these are normal concerns. Actually, the relationship between partners often deepens after surgery. Through sharing of difficulties, partners often become closer emotionally and sexually. For the woman who is single, mastectomy should not interfere with forming sexual relationships or marriage.

Depression is quite common following breast surgery. Within several months, however, most women adjust to their situation. If you continue having difficulties, you may wish to ask your doctor for a referral to a therapist. Many women are relieved to discuss their problems with former mastectomy patients. Reach to Recovery, a national program sponsored by the American Cancer Society, offers women the opportunity to talk on a one-to-one basis with a former mastectomy patient. (See Readings and Resources.) Upon authorization by your surgeon, a Reach to Recovery volunteer can visit you in the hospital. She will give you a Reach to Recovery manual which has useful information about clothes, exercises, and suggestions for bra comfort. You will also receive a temporary breast form (prosthesis), a list of where to purchase breast forms, and information for you and your family.

Aftercare

A day or two after surgery, many hospitals offer exercise courses with trained nurses and, at times, Reach to Recovery volunteers. It is very important to do these exercises both in the hospital and at home. Along with these exercises, you may wish to locate a post-mastectomy exercise program in your community. (Be sure to get your doctor's approval before starting any type of program.) After recovery, your surgery should not interfere with activities such as driving, swimming, playing golf, writing, or sewing. In fact, your doctor will encourage you to resume your former activities after your surgery heals.

Until recently, it was very difficult for post-mastectomy women to locate specialty shops. Lingerie manufacturers have designed special bras and pads that are now available in major department stores and specialty shops throughout the country. After your surgery heals, be sure to be fitted by an expert corsetiere.

Breast reconstruction after mastectomy is gaining favor with some surgeons. After surgery, it is possible in *some* cases for a plastic surgeon to rebuild a breast by implanting a synthetic material under the skin of the chest wall. Other surgeons feel that inserting an implant may hide further breast cancer should it develop. Secondly, a breast reconstruction is expensive (about the same as a mastectomy) and it doesn't look or feel like a natural breast. Whether or not to have your breast reconstructed depends on the condition of your chest wall tissues, the amount of breast cancer — and of course — how badly you want an artificial breast.

☐ PROGNOSIS AND CHECKUPS

Studies show that — more than anything else — the amount of cancer found at diagnosis determines prognosis. While prognosis does vary from woman to woman and from hospital to hospital, lower stage cancers have a much more favorable prognosis than higher stage cancers. For example, the survival rate for Stage I's after mastectomy is about 85 percent. This means that five years after treatment, about 85 percent of all women will be alive. Stage II's are about 65 percent; Stage III's, 45 percent; and Stage IV's are less than 10 percent. Various factors affect prognosis after treatment.

Even so, most cancer specialists agree that at least a ten-year cancer-free period is necessary before there can be any strong hope of cure.

Regular checkups are a must for women with a history of breast cancer. After treatment, ask your doctor how often to schedule your checkup exams. Also, find out the best method of breast self-examination. Of course, if you develop any abnormal symptoms between visits, see your doctor promptly.

Generally, these checkups include thorough gynecologic physical exams, Pap tests, and other laboratory tests. These checkups are essential, so be sure to keep your appointments. These exams enable doctors to provide treatment at the earliest possible time for any condition requiring further treatment.

☐ SELF-EXAMINATION

Do you examine your breasts monthly for a lump or other change that may be cancer? If you haven't up until now, start making it a lifetime habit to do breast self-examination once a month. Before the menopause, examine your breasts every month right after your menstrual period, when your breasts are least swollen and easiest to examine. After the menopause, you may examine your breasts at any time during the month. Many women find the first of the month easiest to remember. After hysterectomy, consult your doctor for the best time. If you discover a breast lump or other changes, see a doctor right away.

Also, be sure your doctor examines your breasts at every exam and instructs you in the method of breast self-examination. If your doctor does not do breast exams, find one who does.

How to examine your breasts

While bathing, do a quick check when hands glide easily over wet, soapy skin.

Check for any lump, hard knot, or thickening.

Arms at sides, look at your breasts before a mirror.

Arms up, look for any change in the size or shape of your breasts, any swelling, dimpling of the skin, or changes in the nipple.

Lie down. Put a pillow under your left shoulder and your left hand under your head.

Fingers flat, use your right hand to check your left breast.

Begin at "A" and follow the arrows, feeling gently for a lump or thickening.

Now examine your other breast.

Squeeze the nipple of each breast. Check for any clear or bloody discharge.

(Adapted from the American Cancer Society, 1978.)

267

21

MENOPAUSE

In a society that idolizes youth and good looks, menopause doesn't have such a good rating. Myths prevail about depressed, hard-to-live-with, exhausted women. Drug manufacturers make matters worse by promoting this image in their advertisements for the medical journals. Typically, these ads portray a victimized middle-aged man standing next to a drab and tired-looking woman. One ad for estrogen replacement therapy states: "For the menopausal symptoms that bother him most." In other ads, children and friends are victimized as well. Unfortunately, our ideas about menopause are frequently formed from ads such as these.

The truth is that menopause is a positive or at least neutral experience for many women. And, for women experiencing difficulties, the solutions don't always have to be drastic. By knowing what to expect and what to do, you can make matters a lot easier for yourself. So, here are the real facts to help you deal with this phase of your life.

☐ MENOPAUSE

Menopause is more than just the end of menstrual periods and reproduction. This makes it sound like an abrupt event or a dramatic change of life. The truth is, menopause is usually just the final stage of a *very* gradual process.

Around the age of 25, the ovaries gradually begin producing less estrogens. (Estrogens have a variety of important

269

effects on a woman's body, including regulation of the menstrual cycle.) Somewhere between the ages of 45 and 55—occasionally earlier or later—the ovaries significantly slow down their activities. Monthly ovulation, or release of an egg from the ovary, diminishes to perhaps once every two months, then to once every six months and so on. As a result, menstrual bleeding becomes irregular since the ovaries are no longer producing enough estrogens to maintain monthly menstrual periods.

As menopause approaches, menstrual periods usually become scantier, shorter, and farther apart. In a few women bleeding becomes heavier for a time. Though some women stop menstruating quite suddenly without symptoms, most women experience several years of irregular periods. At some point, menstrual periods finally stop and menopause occurs. But well past the menopause, the adrenal glands and other body tissues continue to produce small amounts of estrogens even though the ovaries are no longer doing so.

In addition to natural menopause during the forties and fifties, there are other types of menopause. For example, in a few women, menopause occurs prematurely as a result of ovarian disease. When this happens, symptoms gradually begin as early as age 25 and menopause occurs before age 40. Also, there is such a thing as surgical menopause. Right after removal of both ovaries, menstrual periods stop and menopause usually occurs rather abruptly. Radiation therapy to the ovaries or nearby tissues can have the same effect.

Hysterectomy (surgical removal of the uterus) will *not* bring on the menopause unless both ovaries are removed in addition to the uterus. Both ovaries—or even one ovary—can produce estrogens whether or not the uterus is present. However, when younger women must have both ovaries removed or treated with radiation therapy, doctors often prescribe estrogen replacement therapy to prevent abrupt and severe menopausal symptoms.

After your menopause (technically, twelve months after your last menstrual period), you can stop using birth control. Up until then, it is essential to use regular contraception to avoid unplanned (usually more complicated) pregnancies. For during this time — even though your menstrual periods are coming infrequently — you are still ovulating and pregnancy is still possible. Just because you may be having an occasional hot flash, for example, does not mean it is safe to have sex without birth control. Believe it or not, women in their fifties can and do get pregnant. For women approaching the menopause, the safest methods of birth control are the diaphragm or the condom with foam. Another safe method is, of course, sterilization. But the IUD and the birth control pill are out for women over age 40. The IUD can cause irregular vaginal bleeding and the Pill can cause blood clots and heart attacks, especially in women over age 40.

□ SYMPTOMS

If the end of menstruation was the only result of decreased estrogen levels, few women would complain of symptoms or seek medical advice. But low estrogen levels can definitely cause two problems: the notorious hot flashes and vaginal dryness and inelasticity.

In the case of hot flashes, about half of all women experience them around the time of their menopause. In a hot flash, a momentary wave of heat spreads from the chest to the neck and head. It is usually accompanied by patchy flushing and perspiration. Though some women are constantly plagued by flashes, most women have them only occasionally. Moreover, they are especially common during sleep, often resulting in restlessness, fatigue, and irritability. The worst thing about flashes is that they can cause discomfort and embarrassment. Yet they are harmless, temporary, and disappear altogether within a year or so. While doctors do know that estrogen replacement therapy gets rid of hot flashes, this problem also eventually subsides without treatment.

The other symptom distinctly characteristic of the menopause is vaginal dryness and inelasticity, medically known as "vaginal atrophy." Generally, ten or so years after menopause, the vagina becomes less elastic; its lining gets thinner; and vaginal secretions and lubrication decrease. When vaginal atrophy is severe, it can cause itching, burning, and pain during intercourse. Fortunately, most women never develop this problem very severely. In fact, women with active sex lives before menopause may not even be aware of having it. It seems that many women — freed from menstrual periods, the fears of pregnancy, and the anxieties of childrearing — often find sexual fulfillment during this time. When vaginal atrophy is severe, it can be helped with estrogen replacement therapy. But a water-soluble lubricant such as K-Y jelly can also help and is certainly worth the try.

According to most medical experts, hot flashes and vaginal dryness are the *only* physical signs distinctly characteristic of the menopause, other than the end of menstrual periods. The cluster of symptoms including moodiness, nervousness, crying spells, weakness and fatigue seem to be related more to a woman's emotional make-up rather than hormonal status. Menopause can be a difficult time for even the most stable woman. In a society that emphasizes youth, good looks, and sensuality for everyone, aging and loss of reproduction can be a stunning blow. Moreover, between the ages of 40 and 50 a woman is likely to lose her father and later her mother. If married, her children may leave home for college or marriage; if her husband is a failure she has to face this realization; if he is successful he is frequently away from home. For the woman who has no family, the menopause marks the end of any childbearing possibility. And the woman who has not met her career aspirations has to face this realization also.

All of these losses are real and, to varying extents, distressing to most women. Some depression normally accompanies these adjustments. Most women are able to deal with these changes by talking things over with a close friend, a sympathetic husband, or by joining a rap group at a women's center or a community center. Other women may need help from a therapist. If you need emotional support at this time, you may wish to ask your doctor for a referral to a therapist.

☐ CARDIOVASCULAR DISEASE AND OSTEOPOROSIS

Quite a few doctors believe that estrogens also have an important effect on the cardiovascular system (heart and blood vessels) and bone metabolism. But not all doctors agree on this. In fact, some of the sharpest medical controversy concerns the use of estrogen replacement therapy for the prevention and treatment of these problems.

One claim is that estrogen therapy can prevent or delay atherosclerotic cardiovascular disease (heart attack and stroke, for example). Studies show that cardiovascular disease is rare in young menstruating women. Up to age 40, it is at least twenty times more common in men than women in the United States. When it occurs in menstruating women the major risk factors appear to be: cigarette smoking; diabetes; high blood pressure; and/or a high amount of fat (such as cholesterol) in the blood stream. The gap narrows in the 50s and after age 60, women catch up with men. Could it be that estrogens provide some protection to premenopausal women, protection that declines after the menopause?

If estrogens do have an effect on cardiovascular disease, it may be for the worse. Recent evidence shows that estrogens in the form of birth control pills, increase the likelihood of heart attacks in premenopausal women, especially those over age 40. In another study of men with previous heart attacks, low doses of estrogens did not prevent a repeat attack and high doses actually increased the likelihood of another attack.

The most controversial claim for estrogen therapy concerns its use to prevent and treat osteoporosis — the thinning and weakening of the bones. (Contrary to what some people imply, osteoporosis is *not* simply due to the loss of calcium from the bones. Bone thinning is the result of too little bone per volume of tissue.) Far more common in women than men, osteoporosis afflicts about one out of four women by age 75. Symptoms include: backaches; brittle, easily fractured bones (especially hip and lower forearm); a shortening or bending of the spine (the so-called dowager's hump); and the loss of height (generally one to two inches, but as much as six inches). Studies have associated osteoporosis with lowered estrogen levels because it is more common after the menopause and it develops sooner and more severely in women whose ovaries are surgically removed. Yet osteoporosis occasionally occurs in young women with normal estrogen levels. Why some women develop osteoporosis and others don't is unknown. Low estrogen levels are only one factor that tend to promote bone loss. A variety of other medical conditions are also known to cause thinning of bones.

What about the use of estrogen replacement therapy for osteoporosis? While it seems to relieve the pain of osteoporosis in some women—at least temporarily—its value is uncertain since the pain often stops even without treatment. Nevertheless, the most common use of long-term estrogen therapy is for preventing osteoporosis. While current evidence says that estrogen therapy can slow down the progress of osteoporosis, it will *not* stop it completely. And once the bones become thin, doctors simply don't know how to reverse the process. Right now, it seems that the best way to prevent and slow down the process of osteoporosis is a program of proper diet and physical exercise.

☐ ESTROGEN REPLACEMENT THERAPY

As a result of an enormous promotional campaign in the 1960s, millions of women were promised the fountain of youth in a bottle of estrogen pills. The slogan "feminine forever"—also the title of a book that helped spark the estrogen boom—sums up that promise. In fact, estrogens were said to prevent everything from wrinkles to depression. Millions of women swallowed the story along with the pills. But the dream of femininity through a bottle of estrogen has turned into a nightmare for all too many women. For instead of maintaining youth and health, there is mounting evidence that estrogen replacement therapy may actually lead to cancer and other complications.

Since 1975 several groups of researchers have reported that women who take estrogen therapy are anywhere from four to fifteen times more likely to develop cancer of the endometrium (lining of the uterus) than women who do not. Although these reports have not gone unchallenged, most doctors and researchers support the relationship between estrogen therapy and cancer of the endometrium. In 1976 one other study raised the possibility that estrogen users are at higher risk than nonusers for developing breast cancer. But this last study needs to be confirmed by other researchers.

There are also other known hazards of estrogen use. Such side effects as vaginal spotting or profuse bleeding, nausea, abdominal bloating or cramping, breast tenderness, and fluid retention are not uncommon. Postmenopausal bleeding can be especially worrisome since it can also signal cancer. And to rule out cancer, a diagnostic D and C is necessary.

Despite all these problems, a few doctors and many women still believe that menopause is a hormone-deficiency disease, requiring long-term supplemental estrogen. Most medical experts, however, maintain that menopause is not an illness, but a normal phase of life, and that most women do not need estrogen therapy to cope with their symptoms.

The conclusion seems to be that if you can do without hormone replacement, skip the estrogens. (Less than 20 percent of all women have symptoms severe enough to warrant estrogen therapy.) If you and your doctor feel you need them, take estrogens — but only under careful medical supervision and for the shortest period of time. Here are some general guidelines:

- Do you have hot flashes, vaginal atrophy, or osteoporosis? If not, you should not take estrogen replacement therapy. According to medical researchers, flashes and vaginal atrophy are the *only* menopausal symptoms that estrogens can cure. Estrogen therapy also seems to relieve the pain — at least temporarily — of osteoporosis. But right now there is a lot of debate about the relation between estrogens and osteoporosis.

- Don't take estrogens until you carefully weigh what they can do *for* you against what they can do *to* you. For example, are your hot flashes incapacitating or can you learn to live with them? Remembering that your flashes are temporary may ease matters. If you still have your uterus, be careful. (If you have had a hysterectomy, cancer of the endometrium is no longer a concern.)
- If both you and your doctor decide you need estrogen therapy, your doctor should first take a careful medical history and perform a thorough gynecologic physical exam. (See Table 15.) Before your doctor gives you a prescription for estrogen replacement therapy, ask about the risks and benefits of using it. Because of a 1976 ruling by the Food and Drug Administration, drug manufacturers now provide patient brochures with all estrogen prescriptions. This brochure explains how estrogens work, who can use them, what side effects they may have, and what health problems may be related to their use. Read it carefully and consult your doctor if you have questions.
- If you can take estrogens, request the lowest effective dose. According to the Food and Drug Administration, the least hazardous estrogen regimen appears to be: the *lowest* effective dose for the *shortest* possible time. Estrogens are usually taken in a cyclic fashion: three weeks with estrogens followed by one week without them. Research studies show that cancer is more likely to develop in women taking high doses of estrogens and in women taking estrogens for long periods of time.
- If you have only vaginal dryness, ask your doctor about estrogen cream or suppositories (applied to the vagina). So far, local treatment seems to be safer than pills, even though estrogens are also absorbed into the blood stream. This means that creams *may* cause the same side effects as pills although they are less likely to do so. But don't use them until you consider your alternatives.
- If bleeding occurs (termed "withdrawal bleeding"), it

TABLE 15. Contraindications: Who Should Not Use Estrogen Replacement Therapy

Certain women should not use estrogen replacement therapy since it may produce serious complications. Others may be able to do so under close medical supervision only. Whether you can use estrogen therapy is based on your medical history and a gynecologic physical exam. Check this list to see if you have a medical history of any of the following conditions.

WHO SHOULD NOT USE ESTROGENS

Cancer of the breast or reproductive system
Known or suspected pregnancy
Unusual vaginal bleeding that has not been diagnosed by a doctor
Blood clots in the legs, lungs, or elsewhere in the body
Stroke
Heart attack
Chest pain on exertion (angina pectoris)

WHO MAY BE ABLE TO USE ESTROGENS UNDER
CLOSE MEDICAL SUPERVISION ONLY

Family history of breast cancer
Benign breast disease (fibrocystic disease, breast lumps, or an abnormal mammogram)
Mothers who took DES during pregnancy
Elective surgery planned in next four weeks
High blood pressure
Gallbladder disease
Fibroids of the uterus
Liver disease
Asthma
Kidney disease
Epilepsy
Migraine

generally begins toward the end of the week without estrogens. If you develop vaginal bleeding at any other time, call your doctor promptly.

• If you experience any cardiovascular symptoms while using estrogens, see your doctor immediately: chest pain or shortness of breath; coughing up blood; severe pain in the leg or arm; dizziness, fainting, severe headaches; or changes in vision. These could be signs of real trouble.

- During estrogen therapy, see your doctor regularly, every six to twelve months. If more than a year goes by, ask your doctor about a trial period without estrogens. If your symptoms don't reappear, *stop* taking estrogens. If you still need estrogens, ask your doctor about a lower dose.

☐ **HEALTH CARE CHECKUPS**

If you are past your menopause, have regular health care checkups. How often you need to have checkups varies from woman to woman. If you use estrogen replacement therapy, see your doctor regularly every six to twelve months. Usually all other women should have a checkup once a year. But ask your doctor how often to schedule your exams.

Have regular checkups that include a careful medical history and thorough gynecologic physical exam. (See Chapter 1, Health Care Checkups.) Make sure your exam includes a Pap test, measurement of blood pressure, and a breast exam. (If your doctor doesn't do breast exams, find one who does.) The best thing about the Pap test is its ability to detect the early cervical conditions, dysplasia and very early cancer. These symptom-free conditions are almost 100 percent curable if treated early. But the Pap test is not nearly as effective in detecting abnormal cells of the endometrium (lining of the uterus). For this reason, more and more doctors now use endometrial aspiration. In this diagnostic test—a screening test for women at "high-risk" for developing cancer of the endometrium—cells from the endometrium are safely and painlessly removed for laboratory study. If—according to your doctor—you are at *high* rather than *low* risk for developing endometrial cancer, your doctor may recommend this screening test.

Checkups are essential during the menopausal years. Of course, if you develop any abnormal symptoms between checkups, such as abnormal vaginal bleeding or a breast lump, see a doctor promptly. Whatever you do, don't wait to see if your symptom goes away by itself.

GLOSSARY

abdominal cavity. The body cavity that contains most of the digestive organs and the spleen. It is bound by the diaphragm above and the pelvic cavity below.

abortion. Premature termination of pregnancy. Pregnancy may terminate spontaneously from natural causes (natural abortion or miscarriage) or from a medical procedure (induced abortion).

adenosis. Tissue normally present in the cervical canal that extends into the vagina.

adrenal glands. Two small endocrine glands — one located above each kidney — that secrete hormones essential for normal body functioning.

amenorrhea. Lack of menstrual periods. Amenorrhea can be either primary (failure to menstruate by about age 16) or secondary (absence of menstrual periods for longer than three months in already menstruating women).

amniotic sac. The membrane that surrounds the fetus during pregnancy. Also called the bag of waters.

anemia. Any condition characterized by a low count of red blood cells and/or a low concentration of hemoglobin in the blood.

anesthesia. A drug that induces loss of sensation. Anesthesia can be limited to a local area of the body (local) or associated with loss of consciousness (general).

angina pectoris. Severe chest pain that is related to exertion and relieved with rest.

antibiotic. Various substances (such as penicillin) produced by certain fungi, bacteria, and other organisms, that stop the growth of other microorganisms.

antibody. Part of the body's natural defense mechanism or immune system. Any of the various proteins found in the blood, other body fluids, or tissues that are manufactured by the body to fight off harmful bacteria, viruses, or other foreign invaders.

anus. External opening of the digestive tract through which fecal material is expelled.

artery. A blood vessel that carries blood away from the heart to other parts of the body.

anteverted uterus. The normal forward tilt of the entire uterus.

arthritis. Inflammation of a joint or joints.

asymptomatic. Without symptoms.

atherosclerotic cardiovascular disease. Narrowing of the arteries by fatty deposits (atherosclerosis). Atherosclerosis is a major forerunner of angina pectoris, heart attack, and stroke.

at risk. People who run a greater chance of developing certain conditions than other people are considered to be "at risk."

bacteria. A broad term that includes microorganisms which, when abnormally present in the body, may cause infection and disease. (Certain bacteria, if present in small numbers, are harmless and beneficial.)

basal body temperature (bbt). The body's lowest normal temperature at rest. For example, the body's temperature immediately upon arising in the morning.

benign. Not cancerous.

bilateral salpingo-oophorectomy. Surgical removal of both Fallopian tubes and ovaries.

biopsy. Removal of a tiny amount of tissue for microscopic examination and diagnosis.

birth control pill. A contraceptive that prevents pregnancy, by the use of hormones.

bladder. The elastic, sac-like organ that holds the urine.

blood pressure. Pressure of the blood within the arteries.

board-certified. A doctor who has completed a hospital residency in a particular specialty (for example, obstetrics and gynecology), passed qualifying exams, and fulfilled other requirements of that specialty board.

bowel. The digestive tube passing from the stomach to the anus that includes the small intestine, large intestine, and rectum.

breast self-examination. A monthly screening exam in which a woman examines her breasts for any lumps or other abnormal symptoms.

calendar method. A method of natural birth control that determines ovulation with the use of a calendar.

cancer. A colony of very abnormal cells that multiply rapidly and have the ability to spread (metastasize) to other parts of the body.

cancer in situ. See Very Early Cancer.

carcinogenic. A cancer-causing substance.

cardiovascular. Involving the heart and the blood vessels.

carrier. A person who transmits a disease without having any symptoms.

cauterization. A type of treatment where tissues are burned and destroyed with an electrical probe.

cell. A microscopic mass of protoplasm that is the basic building unit of all living matter.

cervical canal. Passageway within the cervix that connects the uterine cavity with the vagina.

cervical mucus method. A method of natural birth control that determines ovulation by recognizing changes in the consistency of the cervical mucus. Also called the Ovulation or Billings Method.

cervicitis. Inflammation and/or infection of the cervix.

cervix. Lower portion of the uterus that projects into the upper vagina.

cesarean section. Delivery of a baby by means of a surgical incision through the abdominal wall and uterus.

chancre. A dull-red, hard, painless sore that is the first symptom of primary syphilis.

chemotherapy. Treatment of infectious disease or cancer with chemical substances or drugs.

circumcision. Surgical removal of the foreskin from the penis.

clitoris. The small, cylindric, erectile organ located just above a woman's urethra. It is extremely sensitive to stimulation and is the source of sexual sensation and orgasm.

colposcope. A diagnostic instrument that simply magnifies the surface of the cervix and vagina.

colpotomy. Surgical incision in the upper vagina to enable inspection of the pelvic organs.

complication. A potentially life-threatening side effect of a drug, diagnostic test, or treatment.

conception. Union of a sperm and an egg.

condom. A very thin, strong sheath for covering the penis to prevent pregnancy and the transmission of sexually-transmitted infections.

cone biopsy. See Conization.

congenital. Physical or mental traits present at birth that are either inherited or caused by some adverse prenatal influence.

conization. Surgical removal of abnormal tissue from the cervix and cervical canal. Also called cone biopsy.

contraceptive. Any drug, device, or method used to prevent pregnancy.

contraindication. Any medical condition or circumstance that advises against the use of a certain drug or procedure.

corpus luteum. Ovarian tissue formed from the remains of the ruptured ovarian follicle after ovulation. It is primarily responsible for the hormone progesterone, which prepares the lining of the uterus to receive the fertilized egg.

crabs. A sexually-transmitted infection caused by a parasite that buries its head inside a pubic hair follicle. Also called pubic hair lice or *Pediculosis pubis.*

cryosurgery. A type of treatment where abnormal tissues are frozen and destroyed by a probe.

culdoscopy. Insertion of a pencil-like viewing scope through a small surgical incision in the upper vagina to inspect the pelvic organs.

culture. A laboratory method that incubates a specimen (such as discharge, urine, or blood) in a special laboratory medium to allow any organisms or bacteria in it to multiply and thus be identified.

cyst. Any abnormal sac in the body containing fluid or soft material.

cystitis. Inflammation and infection of the bladder.

d and c. Short for dilation and curettage. In this diagnostic or therapeutic surgical procedure, successively larger rods are used to widen (dilate) the opening of the cervix. A curette, a spoon-shaped instrument, is then introduced into the uterus to remove tissue from the uterine lining.

diabetes. A medical condition in which the body cannot produce enough insulin, causing high levels of sugar in the blood.

diaphragm. A soft rubber (or plastic) dome-shaped device worn over the cervix for the prevention of pregnancy.

dilation and evacuation. A second trimester abortion technique in which the fetal material in the uterus is removed with forceps.

dilation and suction curettage. A first trimester abortion technique in which the cervix is dilated and then the fetal material in the uterus is extracted under suction. (Suction curettage is sometimes used in the early part of the second trimester.)

discharge. Any abnormal drainage or secretion.

diuretic. A medication that stimulates the kidneys to eliminate excess body fluids.

douche. To cleanse and flush out the vagina with a liquid solution that is usually medicated.

dysmenorrhea. Painful or uncomfortable menstrual periods.

Dysmenorrhea can be without any underlying problem (primary) or be the result of a specific pelvic condition (secondary).

dyspareunia. Sexual intercourse that is painful or difficult.

dysplasia. Abnormal changes in the tissues covering the cervix, for example, that *may* go through a series of changes and eventually become cancer.

ectopic pregnancy. Pregnancy that develops outside the uterus, most often in one of the Fallopian tubes.

ectropian. Tissue normally present in the cervical canal that extends onto the cervix.

edema. Excess accumulation of water and other fluids within the body tissues that produces swelling and weight gain.

egg. A woman's reproductive cell; also called an ovum. During the reproductive years, one ovary usually releases one egg each menstrual cycle.

ejaculation. Discharge of semen from the penis at the time of orgasm.

embolus. Any undissolved material (for example, air, fat, blood clot) that travels in the blood stream and blocks a blood vessel.

embryo. The product of conception from the third through the fifth week of pregnancy. During the first two weeks of pregnancy, it is known as the ovum; from the sixth week until birth, the fetus.

endocrine glands. Any of the ductless glands (such as the ovaries, thyroid, and adrenals) that secrete hormones directly into the blood stream which affect other parts of the body.

endometrial aspiration. A diagnostic test that removes cells from the lining of the uterus for microscopic examination.

endometriosis. A pelvic condition in which bits of endometrial tissue grow outside the uterus, often on the surface of the uterus, ovaries, and Fallopian tubes.

endometrium. Tissue lining of the uterus.

epidemic. A disease that affects an unusually high number of people at the same time.

epidemiologist. A scientist who studies disease occurrences in human populations.

estrogens. One of several hormones produced primarily by the ovaries. Estrogens are responsible for the development and maintenance of a woman's secondary sexual characteristics. Synthetic estrogens are also prescribed for various medical situations.

estrogen replacement therapy. Hormonal treatment for menopausal symptoms.

fallopian tube. One of two small passageways that branch from either side of the uterus, through which an egg travels from the ovary to the uterus.

false-negative result. A laboratory result that is really positive but comes out negative. For example, a negative pregnancy test in a woman who is really pregnant.

false-positive result. A laboratory result that is really negative but comes out positive. For example, a positive pregnancy test in a woman who is not really pregnant.

fertile days. The days when ovulation (and pregnancy) is most likely to occur.

fetus. The product of conception from the sixth week to the end of pregnancy.

fibroadenoma. A common type of noncancerous breast tumor composed of fibrous tissue.

fibrocystic disease. A common noncancerous breast condition generally characterized by the presence of multiple small cysts and thickening of breast tissue.

fibroids. Noncancerous growths of the uterus. Also called leiomyomas or myomas.

follicle. Ovarian sac-like structure that contains an egg.

foreplay. Initial stages of sex that prepare both partners for intercourse. As sexual tensions mount, a woman's vagina normally becomes very wet and lubricated and a man gets an erection.

foreskin. The fold of skin covering the head of the penis in uncircumcised men. Also called the prepuce.

genital herpes. A sexually-transmitted infection almost always caused by herpes virus type 2. Herpes virus type 1, best known as the cause of fever blisters and cold sores on or around the lips, occasionally occurs around the genitals as a result of oral sex.

genital warts. Virus-caused growths on the genitals that are usually the result of sexual contact. Also called *Condyloma accuminata.*

genitals. The sexual and reproductive organs. In a woman this includes the vulva, vagina, uterus, Fallopian tubes, and ovaries; in a man, the penis and testes.

gonorrhea. One of the most common sexually-transmitted infections caused by the bacteria, *Neisseria gonorrhoeae.*

gynecology. The branch of medicine that deals primarily with conditions of a woman's reproductive system.

heart attack. Permanent damage to an area of the heart as a result of obstruction in one of the arteries (coronary) that supply blood directly to the heart. Also called a myocardial infarction.

hemoglobin. Substance in the red blood cells that carries oxygen to tissues throughout the body.

hemophilus vaginitis. Bacteria-caused vaginal infection that is usually the result of sexual contact.

hemorrhage. Excessively heavy bleeding that can be either internal or external.

hemorrhoids. Itching or painful swellings of dilated veins at the anus.

hernia. Protrusion of an organ, or part of an organ, through the wall that normally contains it.

herpes virus type 2. See Genital Herpes.

hormone. A chemical substance produced in one organ or body part that travels in the blood stream to stimulate or affect another organ or body part. Synthetic hormones are also prescribed for various medical situations.

hot flash. A menopausal symptom characterized by a momentary wave of heat accompanied by patchy flushing and perspiration, usually involving the upper portion of the body.

hymen. A thin membrane that partially or completely covers the vaginal opening until it is broken by strenuous activity or during sexual intercourse.

hypernatremia. An abnormally high level of salt in the blood stream.

hyperplasia. Excessive growth of cells in the tissues covering the endometrium, for example. Certain types of precancerous hyperplasia *may* go through a series of changes and eventually become cancer.

hypertension. High blood pressure.

hypothalamus. A major control center at the base of the brain that is responsible for various bodily functions and intimately connected with the pituitary gland.

hysterectomy. Surgical removal of the uterus.

hysterosalpingography. X-ray study of the uterus and Fallopian tubes with radiopaque dye.

hysterotomy. A second trimester abortion technique in which the fetal material is removed through a surgical incision in the uterus.

impotence. A man's inability to obtain or sustain an erection of the penis for sexual intercourse.

incompetent cervix. A cervix that is too weak to carry the weight of a pregnancy developing in the uterus. An incompetent cervix widens prematurely and may be responsible for miscarriage after the first trimester of pregnancy.

infection. Invasion of any part of the body with harmful bacteria or other organisms.

infertility. Temporary or permanent inability to produce a baby. In a woman, this means the inability to give birth to a live baby; in a man, the inability to impregnate a woman.

inflammation. Localized heat, redness, swelling, and pain as a result of irritation, injury, or infection.

informed consent. Explanation of a medical procedure and/or treatment, its risks, side effects, and a description of any alternative types of treatment that exist for the patient. Informed consent may be verbal but is usually written; both forms are legally valid.

insemination. Medical introduction of semen into the uterus for the purpose of reproduction. This can be done with the partner's semen (artificial insemination) or with another man's semen (artificial donor insemination).

intravenous. Within a vein or veins.

in utero. Within the uterus; not yet born.

intrauterine device (IUD). A device worn within the uterus to prevent pregnancy.

kidney. One of two bean-shaped organs located on the upper back wall of the abdominal cavity that maintain proper fluid balance and eliminate waste products through the formation of urine.

laparoscopy. Insertion of a pencil-like viewing scope through a small surgical incision in the abdomen to inspect the abdominal and pelvic organs.

laparotomy. Surgical incision in the abdominal wall to inspect the abdominal and pelvic organs.

l.m.p. Abbreviation for "last menstrual period."

lumpectomy. Surgical removal of a breast tumor.

lymph nodes. Numerous gland-like bodies in the lymphatic system which, by acting as a trap or filter for bacteria, pus cells, and even cancer cells, help to localize any condition to the area being drained.

malignant. Cancerous.

mammography. Special X-ray study of the breast that can detect benign breast disease, suspicious areas, and definite breast cancer.

mastectomy. Surgical removal of the breast. Types of mastectomy include: simple or total (removes only the breast); modified radical (removes the breast and surrounding lymph nodes); and radical (removes the breast, surrounding lymph nodes, and underlying pectoral muscles).

masturbation. Stimulation of the genitals, usually to orgasm, by means other than sexual intercourse.

medical history. Questions about the patient's personal and family health.

menarche. The age at which menstrual periods begin.

meningitis. Inflammation of the membranes of the brain or spinal cord.

menopause. Permanent end of menstrual periods and reproduction.

menstrual cycle. The series of uterine and ovarian changes, due to hormonal influences, that occur from the beginning of one menstrual period to the beginning of the next one.

menstrual extraction. A method practiced by self-help feminist groups that aims at avoiding the discomfort or inconvenience of the menstrual period. Just before the period is due a woman or one of her friends inserts a special tube into the uterus that sucks out the lining normally shed during the menstrual period.

menstrual regulation. A method of ending a suspected pregnancy in which the lining of the uterus is extracted under suction within 14 days after the late menstrual period.

menstruation. Periodic discharge of bloody fluid from the uterus as a result of cyclic hormone changes. Also called *menses* or menstrual period.

metastasis. The spread of cancer cells, for example, from one part of the body to another usually by means of the lymphatic system or blood stream.

midcycle. Time in the menstrual cycle when ovulation usually occurs.

mini-laparotomy. A surgical sterilization procedure in which a small incision is made in the lower abdomen to locate and close off the Fallopian tubes. Also called mini-lap.

miscarriage. Loss of pregnancy from natural causes (as opposed to induced abortion) before the 20th week of pregnancy.

mittelschmerz. Midcycle ovulatory pain occurring at the time of ovulation.

monilia. A fungus-caused vaginal infection that can be contracted in any of several ways. Also called *Candida*, vaginal thrush, or yeast infection.

morning-after contraception. A contraceptive agent for midcycle sexual exposure that prevents pregnancy by stopping implantation of a fertilized egg.

motility. The power of spontaneous movement. One of the characteristics of normal sperm is motility; that is, the ability to swim.

myomectomy. Surgical removal of a fibroid from the uterus.

natural birth control. A method of contraception that prevents pregnancy without the use of drugs or devices.

needle aspiration. Fluid removal of cells from a breast lump, for example, for microscopic examination and diagnosis by means of a needle and syringe.

non-gonoccocal urethritis (ngu). Any inflammation of a man's urethra that is not caused by a gonorrhea infection. NGU is nearly as common as gonorrhea and is frequently mistaken for it.

nonmalignant. Not cancerous.

nurse practitioner. A nurse with broad clinical responsibilities who has received training in a special nurse practitioner program.

obesity. Extremely overweight. Technically defined as being 20 pounds over ideal weight.

oncology. The branch of medicine that deals with cancerous and noncancerous tumors. (Oncology is a cancer specialty.)

oophorectomy. Surgical removal of one or both ovaries.

oral contraceptive. See Birth Control Pill.

orgasm. The climax of sexual excitement that can be achieved through sexual intercourse, masturbation, or other sexual play.

osteoporosis. Thinning and weakening of the bones which is the result of too little bone per volume of tissue.

outpatient. A diagnostic test or treatment not requiring hospitalization that can be done in a doctor's office or clinic.

ovary. One of two reproductive glands in a woman that produce egg cells or ova and secrete the sex hormones estrogen and progesterone.

ovulation. Release of an egg from the ovary.

palpation. Physical examination of the internal organs by means of the hands and the fingers to detect for tenderness, hernia, or an unusual mass.

pap test. Laboratory study for detection of abnormal cells from the cervix. Also called the Pap smear.

parasite. An organism that survives in or on a different organism.

pathology. The branch of medicine that deals with abnormal tissue changes and disease states.

pelvic cavity. The lower portion of the abdominal cavity bound by the bony pelvis and containing the uterus, Fallopian tubes, ovaries, bladder, and rectum.

pelvic examination. Physical examination of the internal reproductive organs.

pelvic inflammatory disease. Infection of the uterus, Fallopian tubes, ovaries, and/or pelvic cavity.

penis. A man's external genital organ. It contains the urethra that carries urine to outside the body and ejaculates sperm when erect and sexually stimulated.

peritonitis. Inflammation and/or infection of the pelvic cavity, usually the result of pelvic inflammatory disease that has advanced past the Fallopian tubes.

phlebitis. Inflammation of a vein.

pituitary gland. A small endocrine gland located at the base of the brain. This "master gland" of the body secretes many hormones on its own that control the other endocrine glands.

placenta. The organ that nourishes the growing fetus during pregnancy. After delivery it is called the "afterbirth."

polyp. A small, usually noncancerous growth that dangles on a stalk.

postcoital test. Microscopic examination of the cervical mucus shortly after sexual intercourse to determine its receptivity to sperm.

postmenopausal. Occurring after the menopause.

post partum. Occurring after the delivery of a baby.

precancerous. Any early, abnormal condition that has the ability to go through a series of changes and eventually become cancer.

premature birth. A baby that is born before the 37th week of pregnancy.

premature ejaculation. A man's inability to control his ejaculatory reflex which results in ejaculation almost immediately after intercourse begins.

premenopausal. Occurring before the menopause.

premenstrual tension. A set of physical and emotional symptoms that certain women experience in the week preceding the menstrual period.

prenatal. Occurring before the delivery of a baby.

progestin. A synthetic progesterone-like hormone preparation.

progesterone. A female sex hormone produced by the corpus luteum as a result of ovulation that helps prepare the uterus for reception of a fertilized egg.

prognosis. Prediction regarding the probable course and outcome of a disease.

prolapse. Falling down of an organ due to inadequate muscular and tissue support. For example, a prolapsed uterus that protrudes into the vagina.

prostaglandin labor induction. A second trimester abortion technique in which prostaglandin is injected through the abdomen into the amniotic sac, causing a woman to go into labor and expel the fetus through the vagina.

prostaglandins. Natural or synthetic fat-like substances that resemble hormones.

prostate. The gland that surrounds a man's urethra at the base of the bladder. This gland provides secretions for transport of sperm during ejaculation.

puberty. The age at which a person becomes sexually mature and able to reproduce. In girls, this is usually between 12 and 14 years of age; in boys, 13 and 16 years of age.

pulmonary embolism. Occurs when a blood vessel to the

lung is blocked by an embolus that has usually traveled from a vein in the lower extremities or pelvic cavity.

pus. A creamy yellow fluid, which is the result of an infection, containing white blood cells (one of the body's first defense mechanisms against infection), bacteria, and dead cells.

radiation therapy. Various irradiation techniques — such as X-ray, radium, and cobalt — that are primarily used for cancer treatment.

rectum. The lowest portion of the large intestine that connects the intestine with the anus.

recurrence. The return of a condition or disease after recovery.

retroverted uterus. A backward tilt of the entire uterus toward the rectum. Also called a tipped uterus.

rubin test. A diagnostic test to determine if the Fallopian tubes are open or blocked. This is done by injecting carbon dioxide through the cervical canal, uterus, and Fallopian tubes.

saline labor induction. A second trimester abortion technique in which salt solution is injected through the abdominal wall into the amniotic sac, causing a woman to go into labor and expel the fetus through the vagina. Also called "salting-out."

salpingitis. Inflammation and/or infection of the Fallopian tubes, usually the result of pelvic inflammatory disease that has advanced past the uterus.

scabies. A sexually-transmitted infection caused by a parasitic mite that burrows itself under the skin.

schiller's test. A diagnostic test for abnormal conditions of the cervix and vagina, based on the fact that normal areas stain deeply with iodine solution while abnormal areas do not stain at all.

screening exam or test. An exam or test that detects for early, mild, asymptomatic conditions. For example, the Pap test screens millions of women yearly for the early, asymptomatic stages of cervical cancer.

scrotum. External sac that contains the testes.

second opinion. Judgment from another doctor about the necessity of recommended treatment.

semen. Fluid ejaculated by a man at orgasm that contains sperm and secretions produced by other glands.

semen analysis. Microscopic examination of semen to determine if it is normal or abnormal. Also called a sperm count.

septic abortion. Miscarriage complicated by infection.

sexually-transmitted infection. Any infection that is primarily transmitted by sexual contact. Also called venereal disease.

sickle-cell anemia. A type of hereditary anemia affecting black people in which the hemoglobin has undergone a change in its protein composition.

side effect. An undesirable effect of a drug, diagnostic test, or treatment.

speculum. A metal or plastic instrument shaped like a duckbill that is used during an internal pelvic exam to inspect the cervix and vagina.

sperm. A man's reproductive cell that is produced by the testes.

sterility. Inability to conceive, usually on a permanent basis.

sterilization. Any of several surgical procedures that makes a man or a woman sterile or unable to reproduce.

stilbestrol. A synthetic estrogen used to treat various medical conditions. It is best known for its adverse effects on DES-exposed daughters. Also called diethylstilbestrol or DES.

stillbirth. The birth of a dead baby.

stress incontinence. See Urinary Stress Incontinence.

stroke. A sudden, neurological event that occurs when a blood vessel to the brain is blocked by an obstruction, hemorrhage, or embolus.

suction curettage. See Dilation and Suction Curettage.

suppository. A small, medicated preparation for insertion into the vagina, rectum, or urethra, that melts at body temperature.

sympto-thermal method. A method of natural birth control that combines the temperature and cervical mucus methods.

syphilis. The most potentially devastating sexually-transmitted infection caused by the spirochete *Treponema pallidum.*

temperature method. A method of natural birth control that determines ovulation by one's keeping a chart of the body's temperature at rest.

testis. One of two reproductive organs located in the scrotum that produce sperm cells and secrete the sex hormone testosterone. Also called testicles.

testosterone. A hormone produced mainly by the testes that is responsible for a man's sexual characteristics. Women also produce small amounts of testosterone.

theoretical effectiveness. The effectiveness of a birth control method when used exactly according to directions.

thermography. A diagnostic procedure that detects cancer of the breast by measuring temperature differences within the breast with a Polaroid camera.

thrombophlebitis. Inflammation of a vein complicated by a blood clot.

thyroid gland. An endocrine gland, located at the front of the neck, that secretes hormones responsible for various metabolic activities.

tipped uterus. See Retroverted Uterus.

trichomonas. A parasite-caused vaginal infection that is usually the result of sexual contact.

tubal ligation. A surgical sterilization procedure in which the Fallopian tubes are cut and/or tied.

tumor. An abnormal growth of tissue that grows independently of its surrounding tissues. A tumor can be cancerous or noncancerous.

urethra. Channel that carries urine from the bladder to outside the body.

urinary stress incontinence. Involuntary loss of urine as a result of physical stresses such as coughing, sneezing, laughing, walking, or lifting.

use effectiveness. The effectiveness of a birth control method after human errors, such as forgetting to take a Pill, are considered.

uterus. Hollow muscular organ that is responsible for menstruation; helping transport sperm; holding the fertilized egg; and developing the fetus through the nine months of pregnancy. Also called the womb.

vaccine. Any substance that, once taken into the body orally or by injection, will immunize or protect a person against certain infectious diseases.

vagina. The passage that extends from the uterus to the vulva. Also called the birth canal.

vaginal spermicide. Chemicals in the form of foam, jelly, cream, suppositories, or foam tablets that are inserted into the vagina before intercourse to kill sperm on contact.

vaginismus. Strong, involuntary, painful contractions of the muscles surrounding the lower vagina when sexual intercourse is attempted.

vas deferens. Passageways that carry sperm from the testes to the urethra.

vasectomy. A surgical sterilization procedure in which the sperm-carrying tubes (vas deferens) are closed off.

venereal disease (vd). See Sexually-Transmitted Infection.

very early abortion. An early first trimester abortion technique in which the fetal material in the uterus is extracted under suction.

very early cancer. Growth of cancer cells that involves only the top layer of the cervix, for example. Also called cancer *in situ*.

virus. Any infectious agent that has the ability to cause infection and disease.

vulva. A woman's external sexual organs.

withdrawal. A method of birth control that involves withdrawing the penis from the vagina just before orgasm.

xeroradiography. Special X-ray study of the breast for detecting benign breast disease as well as breast cancer. Also called xeromammogram.

x-ray. A form of radiation that is used in special diagnostic tests such as mammography, barium enema, and xeroradiography, as well as for the treatment of diseases such as cancer.

READINGS AND RESOURCES

GENERAL

Delusions of Vigor. Better Health by Mail. Consumer Reports, January 1979.
    See this excellent report before you consider buying any of the mail-order health products advertised in America's leading magazines and newspapers.

FDA Consumer. Food and Drug Administration.
    Keep your eye on this very informative magazine from the Food and Drug Administration. It will keep you abreast of the FDA's warnings about health issues.

From Woman to Woman. A Gynecologist Answers Questions About You and Your Body. L. Lanson. Alfred A. Knopf, 1977.
    Questions and answers on many areas of gynecology.

Good Housekeeping Woman's Medical Guide. D. Rorvik. Avon Books, 1976.
    Basic, easy-to-understand guide to obstetrics and gynecology.

Healthright, Inc.
175 Fifth Avenue
New York, New York 10010
(212) 674-3660
    Women's health education and advocacy group that publishes pamphlets and a quarterly newsletter in addition to conducting a patient advocacy program.

The People's Pharmacy. A Guide to Prescription Drugs, Home Remedies, and Over-the-Counter Medications. J. Graedon. Avon, 1977.
    Consumer's guide to the risks, benefits, and side effects of drugs.

Includes useful information on drug interactions, birth control, pregnancy, and how to save money on prescription drugs.

Our Bodies, Ourselves. A Book by and for Women. The Boston Women's Health Book Collective. Simon and Schuster, 1976
Pioneer book on women's health care.

The Woman Patient. Medical and Psychological Interfaces. Sexual and Reproductive Aspects of Women's Health Care, Volume 1. M. T. Notman and C. C. Nadelson (Editors). Plenum, 1978.
Very detailed views of the sexual and reproductive aspects of women's health care.

HEALTH CARE: CHOOSING AND USING IT

America's Best Hospitals for Women. E. Kiester. Ladies' Home Journal, January 1976.
This excellent article comes up with the ten best American hospitals and a list of honorable mentions.

American Hospital Association Guide to the Health Care Field. American Hospital Association. See the most recent edition.
State-by-state directory of hospitals that lists the services they offer, accreditation, and other useful information.

The Consumer's Guide to Health Care. F. Chisari, R. Nakamura, and L. Thorup. Little, Brown, 1976.
Concise, informative book on how to choose doctors, hospitals, and community health agencies.

Directory of Medical Specialists. Marquis-Who's Who. See the most recent edition.
State-by-state list of the age, medical education, and professional background of all Board-certified physicians.

Group Health Association of America, Inc.
Communication and Information Department
1717 Massachusetts Avenue, N.W.
Washington, D.C. 20036
Consult this organization for a list of health maintenance organizations in your area. (The Association's standards for membership offer a measure of consumer protection.)

HMO Program
Room 7-39, Parklawn Building
5600 Fishers Lane
Rockville, Maryland 20857
Consult this office for a list of government-certified health maintenance organizations in your area.

HMOs: Are They the Answer to Your Medical Needs? Consumer Reports, October 1974.
In addition to exploring the pros and cons of health maintenance organizations, this report offers guidelines to help consumers choose a good one.

How to Find a Doctor for Yourself. Consumer Reports, September 1974.
Excellent article on how to interpret a doctor's training and credentials.

How to Talk to Doctors. J. Verby and J. Verby. Arco Publishing, 1977.
Practical, entertaining suggestions for better, doctor-patient communications.

Joint Commission on Accreditation of Hospitals
875 North Michigan Avenue
Chicago, Illinois 60611
(312) 642-6061
Consult this organization or the *American Hospital Association Guide to the Health Care Field* for a list of accredited hospitals in your area.

Money Book. S. Porter. Avon Books, 1976.
See the excellent chapter on health that includes tips on health insurance, shopping for health care, and where to get help.

The Rights of Hospital Patients. G. J. Annas. Avon Books, 1975.
Comprehensive, useful guide from hospital admission to discharge, by the American Civil Liberties Union.

Talk Back to Your Doctor. How to Demand (& Recognize) High Quality Health Care. A. Levin. Doubleday, 1975.
Consumer's guide to judging doctors, hospitals, and how to get high quality medical care.

MENSTRUAL CYCLE

The Curse. A Cultural History of Menstruation. J. Delaney, M. J. Lupton, and E. Toth. New American Library, 1977.
Richly documented book for men and women about the misconceptions of menstruation and menopause.

Menstruation. H. C. Maddux. Tobey Publishing, 1975.
Practical guide to menstruation, including prevention and treatment of menstrual problems.

Menstruation and Menopause: The Physiology and Psychology, the Myth and the Reality. P. Weideger. Alfred A. Knopf, 1976.

History, sociology, and psychology of menstruation and menopause, often related to the comments received from 558 women's questionnaires.

The West Point Fitness and Diet Book. J. L. Anderson and M. Cohen. Avon Books, 1977.
Simple and effective exercise program graded by age and sex. Has special chapter on the role of exercise during menstruation, pregnancy, and menopause.

SEXUALITY

American Association of Sex Educators, Counselors, and Therapists
5010 Wisconsin Avenue, N.W.
Washington, D.C. 20016
(202) 686-2523
Consult AASECT for a list of sex therapists and sex clinics in your area.

Eastern Association for Sex Therapists
4 East 89th Street
New York, New York 10028
Consult EAST for a list of well-qualified sex therapists and sex clinics in your area.

For Yourself: The Fulfillment of Female Sexuality. L. G. Barbach. New American Library, 1976.
Sensitive, step-by-step guide to achieving orgasm.

Fundamentals of Human Sexuality. H. A. Katchadourian and D. T. Lunde. Holt, Rinehart and Winston, 1975.
Straightforward textbook on the biological, psychological, and cultural aspects of sexuality.

The Hite Report. A Nationwide Study of Female Sexuality. S. Hite. Dell, 1978.
Provocative, revealing book based on the detailed responses of 3,019 women who answered questionnaires about sex and sexuality.

The Illustrated Manual of Sex Therapy. H. Kaplan. Addison-Wesley, 1976.
Do-it-yourself book on how to enjoy sex more fully if you are not inclined to see a sex therapist.

The Joy of Sex. A Cordon Bleu Guide to Lovemaking. A. Comfort. Simon and Schuster, 1974.
Thoroughly illustrated handbook on how to add zest and variety to sex.

Sex Information and Education Council of the U.S.
List of publications available from:
Sex Information and Education Council of the U.S.
84 Fifth Avenue, Suite 407
New York, New York 10011

The Sexually Healthy Woman. A. Stitt. Grosset & Dunlap, 1978.
Basic, reassuring guide to sex and sexuality.

Understanding Human Sexual Inadequacy. F. Belliveau and L. Richter. Bantam, 1970.
Simple, complete explanation of Masters' and Johnson's medical text, *Human Sexual Inadequacy.* (Masters and Johnson are well-respected sex researchers who have a clinic in St. Louis, Missouri, called the Reproductive Biological Research Foundation where couples go for help.)

SEXUALLY-TRANSMITTED INFECTIONS

Informational Materials on Venereal Disease
For this list of pamphlets and books write:
Center'for Disease Control
Technical Information Services
Bureau of State Services
Atlanta, Georgia 30333

Operation Venus
(800) 523–1885 (toll-free for all states outside of Pennsylvania)
(800) 462–4966 (toll-free in Pennsylvania)
567–6969 (Greater Philadelphia area)
National VD hotline to help people find a place for diagnosis and treatment nearest home.

Sex and Birth Control. A Guide for the Young. E. J. Lieberman and E. Peck. Schocken Books, 1975.
Mostly deals with birth control, but there are several good chapters on sex and sexually-transmitted infections.

STD Fact Sheet. Center for Disease Control.
Order most recent edition for free from:
Center for Disease Control
Technical Information Services
Bureau of State Services
Atlanta, Georgia 30333

Basic statistics on the sexually-transmitted disease (STD) problem in the United States.

Vaginal Health. C. V. Horos, Tobey Publishing, 1975.
Practical guide to sexually-transmitted infections as well as personal hygiene.

VD. The ABC's. J. W. Grover. Prentice-Hall, 1971.
Basic guide to symptoms, diagnosis, and treatment of sexually-transmitted infections.

The VD Book. For People Who Care About Themselves and Others.
J. A. Chiappa and J. J. Forish. Holt, Rinehart & Winston, 1977.
Folksy questions and answers on sexually-transmitted infections, especially gonorrhea and syphilis.

VD Handbook. Montreal Health Press, Inc.
Order for $.35 from:
Montreal Health Press, Inc.
P.O. Box 1000, Station G
Montreal, Quebec
Canada H2W 2N1

Excellent booklet on sexually-transmitted infections, clearly describing their symptoms, diagnosis, treatment, and complications.

BIRTH CONTROL

Association for Voluntary Sterilization, Inc.
708 Third Avenue
New York, New York 10017
(212) 986-3880
National organization that provides information on the medical and legal aspects of sterilization plus referrals to recommended specialists.

The Birth Control Book. H. I. Shapiro. Avon Books, 1978.
Current, very detailed questions and answers about birth control methods, how they work, and their side effects.

Birth Control Handbook. Montreal Health Press, Inc.
Order for $.35 from:
Montreal Health Press, Inc.
P.O. Box 1000, Station G
Montreal, Quebec
Canada H2W, 2N1

Excellent booklet on birth control methods, how they work, and their side effects.

Contraceptive Technology 1978-1979. R. A. Hatcher, G. K. Stewart, F. Stewart, et al. Irvington Publishers, 1978.

Up-to-date, very useful information (sometimes technical) about birth control. Also has chapters on the menstrual cycle and sexually-transmitted infections.

Planned Parenthood Federation of America, Inc.
810 Seventh Avenue
New York, New York 10019
(212) 541-7800

Planned Parenthood offers a variety of reproductive health services — abortion, pregnancy testing, VD, contraception, sterilization, infertility, and related services — in almost every state. Consult the White Pages for the Center nearest you for health services and the above address for a list of their publications.

Sex and Birth Control. A Guide for the Young. E. J. Lieberman and E. Peck. Schocken Books, 1975.

Highly readable, basic book on birth control and sex.

Women and the Crisis in Sex Hormones. B. Seaman and G. Seaman. Bantam Books, 1978.

Provocative look at birth control (and menopause).

ABORTION

The Abortion Controversy. B. Sarvis and H. Rodman. Columbia University Press, 1974.

Reviews the legal, social, medical, and moral problems of the abortion debate.

Abortion: A Woman's Guide. Planned Parenthood of New York City, Inc. Pocket Books, 1975.

Highly readable, sensitive handbook that guides the reader through getting an abortion.

The Birth Control Book. H. I. Shapiro. Avon Books, 1978.

Most questions and answers deal with birth control, but there is a good chapter on all phases of abortion.

Directory of Providers of Family Planning and Abortion Services. The Alan Guttmacher Institute, 1977.

Order for $5.00 from:
The Alan Guttmacher Institute
515 Madison Avenue
New York, New York 10022

State-by-state directory of clinics and hospitals providing birth control and abortion services. (Alan Guttmacher Institute is the research division of Planned Parenthood.)

A Guide to Pregnancy and Parenthood for Women on Their Own.
P. Ashdown-Sharp. Vintage, 1977.
Single women's guide to pregnancy, parenthood, and birth control. Includes useful information about pregnancy tests, abortion, keeping your baby versus adoption or fostering, and finding financial and emotional assistance. (Regardless of the title, all women can benefit from using this book.)

How to Choose an Abortion Facility. National Abortion Federation.
Order this pamphlet for free from:
National Abortion Federation
110 East 59th Street
New York, New York 10022

Planned Parenthood Federation of America, Inc.
For pregnancy testing and/or an abortion, consult the White Pages for the Planned Parenthood Center in your community. Many of these Centers offer pregnancy testing and some perform abortions. If the Planned Parenthood in your area does not perform abortions, they can refer you to a place that does.

Test Yourself for Pregnancy? Consumer Reports, November 1978.
See this excellent report before you consider using a do-it-yourself pregnancy test.

STILBESTROL EXPOSURE

Brink of Tragedy. E. Keiffer. Good Housekeeping, July 1974.
Relates the personal experience of a young woman who developed vaginal cancer as a result of DES exposure.

Questions and Answers About DES Exposure Before Birth. DESAD Project.
Order this pamphlet for free from:
Office of Cancer Communications
National Cancer Institute
Bethesda, Maryland 20014

Stilbestrol Exposure. C. Derbyshire, Boston Hospital for Women, 1976.
Order this pamphlet for $.75 with self-addressed envelope from:
Office of Information Services
Affiliated Hospitals Center, Inc.
Boston, Massachusetts 02115

DES Action, National
Contact their national headquarters for your nearest office:

Long Island Jewish-Hillside Medical Center
New Hyde Park, New York 10040
(212) 343-9222

National volunteer organization that provides information, referrals, and support groups for DES-exposed women and their families.

INFERTILITY

The Adoption Adviser. J. McNamara. Hawthorn Books, 1976.
Current and complete resource about all types of adoptions.

American Fertility Society
1608 Thirteenth Avenue South
Birmingham, Alabama 35205
(205) 933-7222
This national organization concerned with infertility can give you
names of specialists nearest home who provide infertility services.

Infertility. A Couple's Guide to Causes and Treatments. M. Harrison.
Houghton Mifflin, 1977.
Informative discussion about both the medical and emotional aspects of infertility. (The author and her husband were an infertile
couple.)

Infertility. A Guide for the Childless Couple. B. E. Menning. Prentice-
Hall, 1977.
Sound, very thorough advice for the infertile couple.

Resolve, Inc.
P.O. Box 474
Belmont, Massachusetts 02178
(617) 484-2424
National organization serving people affected by infertility. Provides
counseling and information, referrals to recommended specialists,
support groups, and adoption resources. Contact their main office
for the chapter nearest you.

SURGERY

*Every Woman's Guide to Hysterectomy. Taking Charge of Your Own
Body.* D. Jameson and R. Schwalb. Prentice-Hall, 1978.
Personal experience plus sound, basic information provide reassur-
ance for any woman facing hysterectomy.

Ghost Surgery: Standard Operating Procedure. T. Cohen. Harper's Bazaar, July 1978.
A close look at who actually performs surgery in teaching hospitals.

Hysterectomy. B. Anderson. In: *The Menopause Book.* L. Rose, Editor. Hawthorn Books, 1977.
Excellent discussion of the occasions when hysterectomy is necessary and what it includes.

Important Questions to Ask Before You Let Them Operate. Changing Times, February 1979.
In addition to suggesting questions to ask before surgery, this superb report offers guidelines to help consumers choose a good surgeon.

Needless Hysterectomies. M. Cohen. Ladies' Home Journal, March 1976.
Brief account of the hysterectomy controversy.

The New Understanding Surgery: The Complete Surgical Guide. R. E. Rothenberg. New American Library, 1976.
This encyclopedic guide contains straightforward information on problems requiring surgery.

What Every Woman Should Know About Hysterectomy. W. Gifford-Jones, Funk & Wagnalls, 1977.
A practicing gynecologist tells exactly what you need to know before and after hysterectomy.

When Do You Need a Second Opinion? W. A. Nolen. McCalls, April 1979.
Excellent guidelines on when to get a second surgical opinion.

CANCER FACTS

American Cancer Society, Inc.
777 Third Avenue
New York, New York 10017
(212) 371-2900
The American Cancer Society is a national, voluntary organization devoted to programs in cancer research, patient services, and health education. Contact your local office listed in the White Pages or their national headquarters for general cancer information and a list of their publications. Though the American Cancer Society does not have a policy of giving out physician referrals, your local office can give you general advice about what to do and how to locate your own physician.

National Cancer Institute
Office of Cancer Communications
Bethesda, Maryland 20014
(301) 496-6631
The National Cancer Institute is the federal government's principal agency for cancer research and health education. It also provides patient services through its nationwide network of Comprehensive Cancer Centers. You can contact this office for general cancer information and a list of their publications. Also, this office can help cancer patients and their doctors find names and addresses of cancer specialists nearest home.

Preventing Cancer. What You Can Do to Cut Your Risks by up to 50 Percent. E. Whelan. W. W. Norton, 1978.
Practical, everyday ways to reduce the risk of getting cancer.

Primer of Epidemiology. G. D. Friedman. McGraw-Hill, 1974.
Good, basic book about clinical research studies. (For example, the much discussed prospective and retrospective case-control studies.)

What You Need to Know About Dysplasia, Very Early Cancer and Invasive Cancer of the Cervix. C. Derbyshire and R. C. Knapp. National Cancer Institute, 1980.
Order this pamphlet for free in English and/or Spanish from:
Office of Cancer Communications
National Cancer Institute
Bethesda, Maryland 20014

You Can Fight Cancer and Win. J. E. Brody. McGraw-Hill, 1978.
Comprehensive guide to cancer prevention, diagnosis, and treatment by a *New York Times* medical writer. Included in the appendix is a list of nationwide Comprehensive Cancer Centers that provide current information and excellent cancer care.

BREAST CANCER

American Cancer Society, Inc.
777 Third Avenue
New York, New York 10017
(212) 371-2900
Contact your local office listed in the White Pages or their national headquarters for general cancer information and a list of their publications. Though this agency does not have a policy of giving out physician referrals, your local office can give you general advice about what to do and how to locate your own doctor.

The Complete Breast Book. M. Storch and L. May. Good Housekeeping, February 1979.

Short, informative article covering breast development, daily breast care, benign breast disease, and breast cancer.

National Cancer Institute
Office of Cancer Communications
Bethesda, Maryland 20014
(301) 496–6631

Contact this office for general cancer information and a list of their publications. Also, this office can help cancer patients and their doctors find names and addresses of cancer specialists nearest home.

The Complete Book of Breast Care. R. E. Rothenberg. Ballantine Books, 1976.

Practical guide to breast development, daily breast care, benign breast disease, and breast cancer.

First, You Cry. B. Rollin. New American Library, 1977.

Fast-moving, sensitive account of this NBC news correspondent's encounter with breast cancer.

Post-Mastectomy: A Personal Guide to Physical and Emotional Recovery. W. A. Winkler. Hawthorn Books, 1976.

Practical advice about what to do after breast surgery, written by a woman who has been through it.

Reach to Recovery Foundation
44 East Fifty-Third Street
New York, New York 10022
(212) 586–8700

National organization sponsored by the American Cancer Society that offers physical and emotional support to mastectomy patients.

Three Weeks in Spring. J. H. Parker and R. B. Parker. Houghton Mifflin, 1978.

One family's dealings with breast cancer. (This skillfully-written story has a happy ending.)

What We Now Know About Breast Cancer. W. A. Nolen. McCalls, July 1978.

Excellent review of current methods of diagnosing and treating breast cancer.

Why Me? What Every Woman Should Know About Breast Cancer to Save Her Life. R. Kushner. New American Library, 1977.

Very comprehensive book about breast cancer, covering its causes, diagnosis, treatment, and rehabilitation, written by a woman who has been through it.

You Can Fight Cancer and Win. J. E. Brody. McGraw-Hill, 1978.

Mostly deals with cancer in general, but there is a good, brief chapter on breast cancer.

MENOPAUSE

Estrogen Therapy: The Dangerous Road to Shangri-La. Consumer Reports, November 1976.
Good explanation of the early studies associating estrogen replacement therapy with cancer of the endometrium. Also has sound advice for women who choose to use estrogen therapy.

The Menopause Book. L. Rose, Editor. Hawthorn Books, 1977.
Eight women physicians apply their expertise to this sound and very thorough handbook.

Menstruation and Menopause: The Physiology and Psychology, the Myth and the Reality. P. Weideger. Alfred A. Knopf, 1976.
History, sociology, and psychology of menstruation and menopause, often related to the comments received from 558 women's questionnaires.

Passages: Predictable Crises of Adult Life. G. Sheehy. Bantam Books, 1977.
Descriptive analysis of the emotional stages of adult life, often related to 115 case histories.

The Psychology of Women. Volume II: Motherhood. H. Deutsch. Bantam Books, 1973.
Richly-documented study of the needs, social pressures, and personality problems of motherhood by one of Sigmund Freud's disciples. Has a special chapter on menopause.

Love and Sex After Sixty. A Guide for Men and Women in their Later Years. R. N. Butler and M. I. Lewis. Harper & Row, 1977.
Highly-readable, practical guide to the social, medical, and psychological problems of sex.

Women and the Crisis in Sex Hormones. B. Seaman and G. Seaman. Bantam Books, 1978.
Provocative look at menopause (and birth control).

INDEX

Abdomen
  examination of, 12, 14
Abortion, 167-190
  aftercare of, 188-189
  alternatives to, 168, 173, 178
  assistance in getting, 174-
    176
  and birth control, 99, 115,
    125, 144, 161, 162
  and diagnosis of pregnancy,
    169-172, 178, 182
  facilities for, 176-180
  feelings about, 172-173, 189-
    190
  risks of, 82-84, 186
  types of, 180-188
Abstinence. *See* Sexual inter-
    course
Adoption, 215-216
Amenorrhea. *See* Menstruation,
    absence of
American Association of Sex
    Educators, Counselors, and
    Educators, 48, 302
American Cancer Society (ACS),
    251, 308, 309
  and assistance in locating
    doctors, 246-247, 258
  and Pap tests, 13
  and Reach to Recovery, 264
  and warning signals of cancer,
    235-236
American Fertility Society, 205,
    307
Anemia
  iron-deficiency, 110, 118
  sickle-cell, 186
Antibiotics
  in bladder infections, 225
  in cervicitis, 77, 213
  in pelvic inflammatory disease,
    84
  in VD, 52, 57, 61, 69, 71, 72

Artificial insemination, 214-215
Association for Voluntary Sterili-
    zation, 160, 304

Basal body temperature chart
  as infertility test, 210
  as method of birth control,
    145-147
Biopsy
  of breast, 255-256
  of cervix, 77, 230-231, 239.
    See also Conization
  of endometrium, 30, 210
  of vagina, 243
  of vulva, 243
Birth control, 87-165. *See also*
    Breast-feeding; Condom;
    Diaphragm; Douching; In-
    trauterine devices; Morning-
    after IUD; Morning-after
    pill; Natural birth control;
    Oral contraceptives; Sexual
    Intercourse; Sterilization;
    Vaginal spermicides; With-
    drawal
  choosing a method, 89-91
  effectiveness of, 90-91
  during menopause, 270-271
  where to get, 91
Birth defects, 109
Bisexuality, 35
Bladder infection, 75-76
Bleeding, abnormal
  after douching or intercourse,
    85, 238, 243
  after menopause, 238, 277,
    278
  between periods, 30, 80, 85,
    118, 238, 241, 243, 244
Blood clotting disease
  and oral contraceptives, 103-
    105, 223, 271

313